Diabetes Balanced Diet.

Dr. Neal Allan.

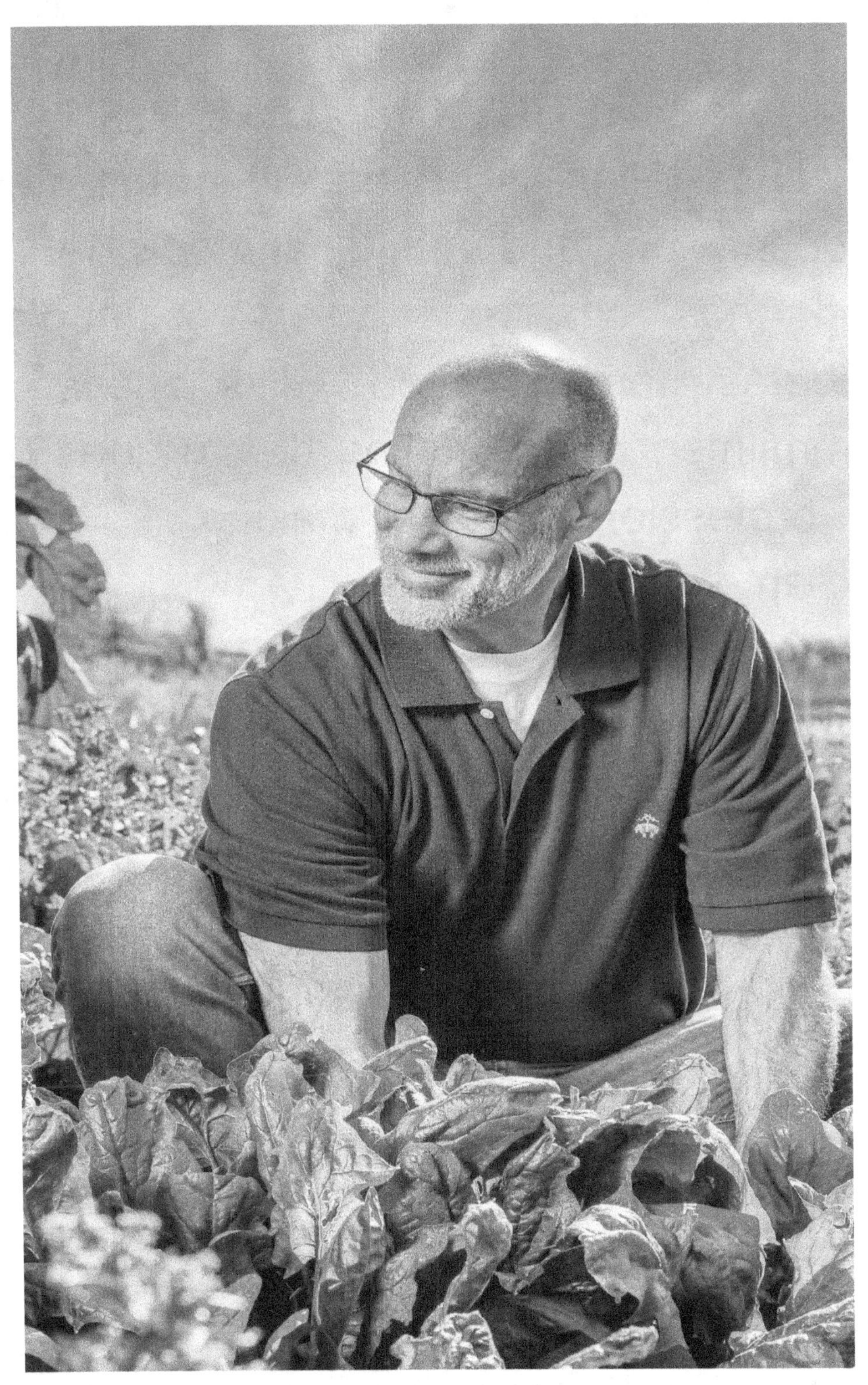

Dr. Neal Allan.

ABOUT THE AUTHOR.

Dr. Neal Allan is a leader in the fields of endocrinology and nutritional medicine, and his work has changed the way people with diabetes are treated. His never-ending commitment to promoting health goes beyond the professional setting, making him an expert and an example.

With a lot of experience taking care of people with diabetes, Dr. Allan brings a unique point of view to the table. Beyond his medical business, he strongly advocates for empowering people to take charge of their health. A creative addition to health publications and community programs, Dr. Allan tries to make a lasting effect on public understanding and education.

His dedication is reflected in the pages of "Diabetes Balanced Diet," a testament to his belief that managing diabetes can be a delicious and satisfying journey. Dr. Neal

Allan's holistic approach, paired with a flair for making informed choices delicious, places him as a leading voice in the quest for lively, healthy living amidst the challenges of diabetes.

CHAPTER ONE.

Understanding Diabetes and Nutrition.

What is diabetes?

Diabetes is a medical disorder caused by high blood glucose, also known as blood sugar. Glucose is your body's main energy source. Glucose originates from meals, yet the body may also manufacture it.

When the pancreas secretes the hormone insulin, glucose is absorbed and used by your cells for energy more readily. Diabetes is caused by either inadequate insulin synthesis or inappropriate insulin use by the body. After that, glucose remains in your circulation rather than entering your cells.

Diabetes raises the risk of damage to the kidneys, nerves, heart, and eyes. There is a connection between diabetes and several cancers. You may be able to reduce your chance of getting diabetes-related health issues if you take action to prevent or manage your diabetes.

37.3 million people in the US have diabetes. Moreover, a higher proportion of people are ignorant of the fact that they are at a considerable risk of developing prediabetes or developing Type 2 diabetes in the future. Though Type 2 diabetes is usually considered to occur after prediabetes, Type 2 diabetes may be prevented or delayed with major lifestyle changes.

All forms of diabetes affect how well the body produces and uses insulin. The hormone insulin, which is produced by the pancreas, helps your cells store and use the energy from meals. Blood glucose accumulates in diabetics but is not absorbed by the cells. Your body isn't getting enough energy as a consequence. Additionally, when too much glucose is circulated throughout the body, cells are harmed along the way.

Diabetes increases the risk of heart attack and stroke, but it may also damage kidneys, eyes, and nerves.

Types of Diabetes:

There are several intricate and little-known causes of diabetes. Even though food does not cause diabetes, it is a part of the care strategy for the illness.

There are three main types of diabetes:

1. Type 1 diabetes:

The pancreas either produces too little or none at all. Type 1 diabetes is an autoimmune disease that often begins in infancy. The start is sudden. Type 1 diabetes affects just 5.7% of people with diabetes who use insulin. Changes in diet and lifestyle may help control this condition, but they cannot stop it.

2. Type 2 diabetes:

The pancreas produces insulin, but the body either doesn't utilize it or doesn't use enough of it. Type 2 usually advances slowly. Approximately 89% of individuals with this kind of diabetes are considered overweight or obese based on their body mass index (BMI). Other risk factors include an older age, impaired glucose metabolism, inactivity, and a history of gestational diabetes.

• Diabetes during pregnancy:

The body produces inadequate amounts of insulin during pregnancy, which is the cause of this illness. It's thought that other hormones could interfere with insulin's ability to function. Gestational diabetes usually goes away once the baby is delivered. However, women with this kind of diabetes have a higher chance of developing kind 2 diabetes later in life.

How to Reduce Your Chance of Diabetes.

Type 2 diabetes may be prevented or delayed by making dietary changes, increasing your level of physical activity, and losing a certain amount of weight if your BMI places you in the overweight or obese group. By doing these things, the likelihood of diabetic complications is reduced. Visit a registered dietitian nutritionist to learn how to change your way of living and reduce your chance of developing Type 2 diabetes.

Gestational diabetes.

One kind of the illness that might arise is diabetes associated with pregnancy. This kind of diabetes almost always goes away once the baby is delivered. Conversely, having gestational diabetes raises your chance of developing type 2 diabetes later in life. Sometimes diabetes during pregnancy is mistaken for type 2 diabetes.

Before diabetes.

Patients with prediabetes have higher blood glucose levels than healthy individuals, but not high enough to be considered type 2 diabetes. If you have prediabetes, you have a higher chance of developing type 2 diabetes later in life. Additionally, you have an increased risk of heart disease in comparison to those with normal glucose levels.

Various types of diabetes:

A less common variant of the condition called monogenic diabetes is caused by a single gene mutation. Diabetes may also be brought on by conditions like pancreatitis or cystic fibrosis that damage the pancreas, as well as after pancreatic removal surgery.

Signs, Symptoms, and Testing:

Diabetes may lead to a number of symptoms, including impaired circulation, which can cause tingling or numbness in the hands and feet, excessive thirst, weight loss without conscious effort, exhaustion, blurred vision, and recurring infections or diseases. Do not delay in seeking medical attention if you experience any of these signs. You may need to have one of the following tests to check for diabetes:

• Plasma glucose after fasting.

This test calculates the amount of glucose present in a blood sample taken from a fasting person (usually meaning that the individual has not eaten in eight to twelve hours).

•A1C Test:

finds the person's average blood glucose range during the preceding two to three months. This test shows the quantity of glucose that sticks to the red blood cell.

• Test for Oral Glucose Tolerance:

The results of this test show how the body consumes glucose over an extended period of time. This test is performed by a medical specialist after an overnight fast. The patient is given a high-glucose beverage after the blood is drawn, and further blood draws may be performed every hour for up to three hours after the beverage is consumed.

Managing Blood Sugar Levels:

To assist you in controlling your blood glucose, a registered dietitian nutritionist will work with you and other members of the medical team.

levels and minimize the possibility of future issues if you have been identified as having diabetes. You and your care team may work together to achieve the following goals:

• Keeping blood glucose levels as close to normal as is practical will help prevent or minimize complications.

• Keeping blood pressure within normal ranges. trying to reach the ideal cholesterol range.

People with Type 1 diabetes need to take insulin injections every day or use insulin pumps. People with Type 2 diabetes may control their blood sugar levels with diet, exercise, and, in certain circumstances, a combination of medication and insulin injections.

Tips for Healthy Eating to Help Control Diabetes.

• Cutting down on the quantity of meals and drinks that have added sugar.

• Selecting smaller portions spread out throughout the day.

• Choosing whole grains, fruits, and vegetables can help you increase the amount of carbohydrates in your diet while reducing your intake of processed carbohydrates.

•Eating a variety of fruits and vegetables, healthy grains, lean protein sources, and dairy products that are low in fat or fat free on a regular basis.

•Emphasizing the use of healthy fat sources including avocados, nuts, seeds, and olive and canola oil while reducing the consumption of saturated fat.

•If you choose to drink, keep your intake to a minimum. Ensure that you consult your healthcare provider about it.

• Using less salt.

Getting Around the Diabetic Food Scene.

Navigating the diabetic food landscape might seem like a difficult journey, but with the right information and a thoughtful approach, it truly becomes a potent exploration of delicious and nutritious alternatives. To maintain stable blood sugar levels and improve overall health, individuals with diabetes must understand the foundations of diabetic diet. This map will assist you in navigating this area:

1. Accept Unprocessed, Whole Foods.

•Reasons: Because whole meals are rich in fiber, antioxidants, and other nutrients, they provide sustained energy without quickly elevating blood sugar levels.

•How: Make lean meats, fresh produce, whole grains, healthy fats, and whole fruits and veggies your top priorities.

2. Expert Management of Carbohydrates.

•Reasons: Carbohydrates have a direct effect on blood sugar levels. Glycemic control depends on regulating the kind and amount.

•How: Choose complex carbs with a low glycemic index, restrict portion sizes, and distribute your daily carbohydrate consumption.

3. Being Aware of the Glycemic Index (GI).

•The GI indicates the rate at which food raises blood sugar levels. Low-GI foods help maintain stable blood sugar levels because they absorb more slowly.

•How: Prioritize low-GI items in your diet, such as whole grains, legumes, and non-starchy vegetables.

4. Give Lean Proteins Your Highest Concern.

Reasons: Protein decreases the overall impact of meals on glucose levels by increasing satiety and stabilizing blood sugar.

•How: Incorporate items like low-fat dairy, fish, chicken, legumes, and tofu into your diet.

5. Good Fats Are Your Friend.

•The Reason: Healthy fats promote heart health and the preservation of fullness.

•How: Choose foods like avocados, almonds, seeds, and olive oil and minimize your intake of saturated and trans fats.

6. Portion Management Is Essential.

•Reasons: Portion control helps control calories and blood sugar levels.

•How: Use moderation, observe serving sizes, and avoid overindulging.

7. Measure Your Blood Sugar.

•Reasons: Regular observation clarifies the manner in which different diets affect blood sugar levels.

• How: Follow your doctor's monitoring recommendations and adjust your diet as needed.

8. It's Vital to Stay Hydrated.

•Reasons: Getting enough water aids in digestion and supports overall health.

•How: Drink primarily water and avoid sugar-filled drinks as much as possible.

9. Learn How to Interpret Food Labels.

•Why: By carefully reading food labels, you may make educated choices about the quantity of carbs and nutritional content.

•How: Pay attention to the ingredients, serving sizes, and overall carbohydrate content.

10. Get Expert Counsel.

• The Reason: Everybody has unique needs. Individualized guidance is ensured by consulting with licensed nutritionists and other medical specialists.

•How: Consult with medical specialists to design a diet tailored to your individual health goals.

Being informed, cultivating a positive connection with food, and maintaining a delicious and diverse diet are the keys to successfully navigating the food landscape for diabetes. If people have a strong foundation of information and ongoing support, they may confidently adopt a lifestyle that not only controls diabetes but also promotes long-term health and well-being.

CHAPTER TWO.

Creating Good Balance of Nutrition. (Protein, Fats and Carbohydrates)

The ideal ratio of carbohydrates to fat in type 2 diabetes.

People with type 2 diabetes have incorrect blood sugar processing, according to the American Diabetes Association (ADA). Thus, monitoring carbohydrates—which the body breaks down into glucose and elevates blood sugar levels for—can help with diabetes management.

You should be mindful of the kind of carbs you eat. She says that consuming more carbs that are high in nutrients will improve your blood sugar's capacity to regulate and prolong your sensation of fullness. This includes foods like rolled oats, brown rice, and whole-wheat pasta.

The American Diabetes Association states that your exercise level and weight-management goals will determine how much carbs is good for you. You may get help figuring this out from a certified diabetes educator or registered dietitian.

The Centers for Disease Control and Prevention (CDC) usually recommend getting around half of your daily calories from carbs, while the recommended quantity for each person may vary. That comes out to around 200–250 grams per day on a 1,800–2,000 calorie diet, which you may split evenly between your meals.

When meal planning for diabetics, it's important to keep in mind that one dish equals fifteen grams of carbs (CDC).

The Ideal Ratio of Protein in Type 2 Diabetes.
Many type 2 diabetics discover that 20 to 25 percent of their daily calories come from protein, while the appropriate ratio of protein to calories varies from person to person.

The Ideal Macronutrient Ratios for People with Diabetes.

If you have type 2 diabetes, you know how hard it is to keep your blood sugar under control, never mind maintaining the right ratios of carbs, proteins, and fats. Experts go over the best macronutrient ratio for diabetics in this article, along with a simple meal plan example.

When meal planning for diabetics, it's important to keep in mind that one dish equals fifteen grams of carbs (CDC).

The Ideal Fat Ratio for People with Type 2 Diabetes.

According to Kimberlain, it's typically recommended to get 25 to 30 percent of your daily calories from fat.

The Ideal Macronutrient Ratios for People with Diabetes 2.

If you have type 2 diabetes, you know how hard it is to keep your blood sugar under control, never mind maintaining the right ratios of carbs, proteins, and fats. Experts go over the best macronutrient ratio for diabetics in this article, along with a simple meal plan example.

The Ideal Ratio of Protein in Type 2 Diabetes: Aiming for 20 to 25 percent of daily calories to come from protein may help many type 2 diabetics find the optimal fuel, while the appropriate daily consumption varies depending on individual factors.

That is equivalent to 140–184 grams per day, based on the United States National Library of Medicine (NLM).

As per Kimberlain, turkey, beans, poultry, almonds, seeds, and seafood are some of the best sources of protein.

If you get your protein from animal sources, go for thinner cuts.

• Pick lean portions of hog, veal, wild game, and beef.

• Lower the amount of visible fat in meat; • Take the skin off of turkeys and chickens; • Bake, roast, boil, or broil rather than frying proteins; • Serve fish and poultry more often.

• Fiber's Effect on Blood Sugar.

The impact of fiber on blood sugar is a significant consideration for individuals, particularly those managing their diabetes self-management. Diets high in plants include fiber, which is a kind of carbohydrate that the body cannot fully digest. Since fiber usually eludes digestion and doesn't break down into sugar molecules, it has a lot of positive effects on blood sugar levels.

1. Delays Absorption and Digestion: Why It Matters.

This progressive procedure reduces the likelihood of abrupt spikes in blood sugar after meals. 1. High-fiber diets impede the absorption and digestion of nutrients, particularly carbs.

2 Manages the Release of Glucose:
Why It Matters.
Soluble fiber, which is included in foods like fruits, legumes, and oats, creates a gel-like material in the digestive system that decreases the pace at which glucose from carbs enters the bloodstream. This helps to maintain more stable blood sugar levels.

3. Promotes Fullness:
Why It Matters.
Foods rich in fiber tend to be more substantial, which promotes fullness and reduces the likelihood of overindulging.
Maintaining a healthy weight is crucial for the control of diabetes. Being satiated might assist with this.

4. Improves Sensitivity to Insulin:

Studies suggest that a diet rich in fiber may improve insulin sensitivity, making it easier for the body to utilize insulin to regulate blood sugar levels.

Increased insulin sensitivity is beneficial for those with insulin resistance, which is a prevalent cause of type 2 diabetes.

5. Reduces the Glycemic Index:

Why It Matters.

Foods with a lower GI tend to have more fiber.

•Foods with a low glycemic index (GI) absorb more slowly, which causes blood sugar levels to climb more gradually and steadily.

6. Aids in the Management of Weight:

Why It Matters.

• Eating high-fiber foods often requires chewing them for longer periods of time, which slows down eating and allows the body more time to sense fullness.

•Controlling weight is crucial for both treating and preventing diabetes, and this may assist.

7. Sources of Dietary Fiber: Why It Matters.

• Nuts, fruits, vegetables, whole grains, and legumes are excellent sources of dietary fiber.

•One may ensure they are receiving enough soluble and insoluble fiber by include a variety of these items in their diet.

8. Suggestions for Increasing Fiber Intake: Why It Matters.

•Give your digestive system time to adjust by progressively increasing your intake of fiber.

•Drink plenty of water since fiber absorbs water and helps it travel through the digestive system.

To summarize, individuals with diabetes may benefit from understanding the impact of fiber on blood sugar levels. By consuming more foods rich in fiber in their diet, they may help control their diabetes better, promote stable blood sugar levels, and enhance their overall health. As usual, for personalized advice based on their particular situation and health goals, individuals should consult with medical doctors or certified dietitians.

30 Insightful and Delectable Meal Options:

Choosing wholesome and delicious meals is essential for diabetics. Thirty mouthwatering, high-nutrient meals that help keep blood sugar levels steady are listed below:

1. Adobo.

Avocados are a tasty, flexible dietary choice that are rich in fiber and good fats.

2. Salmon.

Because of its high omega-3 fatty acid content, salmon is an excellent source of protein for heart health.

Collard, kale, and spinach greens are rich in essential nutrients and low in carbs.

4. Berries.

Antioxidant-rich low-GI foods include blueberries, strawberries, and raspberries.

5. Greek yogurt-based yogurt.

Because Greek yogurt is low in carbs and strong in protein, it makes a great breakfast or snack.

6. Nuts.

Nuts that are high in healthy fats and have a delicious crunch include pistachios, walnuts, and almonds.

7. Quinoa.

Wholesome whole grain with fiber and protein.

8. Broccoli.

Broccoli is a versatile vegetable with a high fiber content and low carbohydrate content.

9. The kale.

A low-carb option to rice or mashed potatoes.

10. Chia Seeds.

Omega-3 fatty acid and fiber-rich chia seeds make a great addition to smoothies or yogurt.

11. Trimmed Breast of Chicken.

An excellent lean protein option for grilling, baking, and sautéing.

12. Sweet potatoes.

A low-glycemic, healthful alternative to regular potatoes.

13. Asparagus.

Low in carbs and high in vitamins and minerals.

14. Eggs.

An excellent source of protein that may be used into several dishes.

15. Olive Oil.

A great, heart-healthy fat for dressing or cooking.

16. Tomatoes.

Rich in antioxidants and versatile enough to work well in salads or sauces.

17. Tofu.

a source of plant-based protein that works well in a range of dishes.

18. Lettuce.

Because it is low in carbs and high in fiber, cabbage is a healthy choice.

19. Flaxseeds.

Rich in fiber and omega-3 fatty acids, flaxseeds are a great addition to smoothies and cereal.

20. Green Beans.

A low-calorie, high-fiber vegetable that complements many different dishes.

21. Cottage Cheese.

A satisfying snack that is rich in protein and low in carbs is cottage cheese.

22. Brussels Sprouts.

Nutrient-rich vegetable that enhances taste.

23. Garlic.

Improves taste without packing on the calories and may be beneficial to your health.

24. Artichokes.

A delicious, high-fiber vegetable that cooks well on the grill or roasting pan.

25. Bell peppers.

Bell peppers are a vibrant, low-carb addition to stir-fries or salads.

26. Turkey.

A versatile option for lean protein in a range of dishes.

27. Cucumber.

A low-carb and hydrating choice is cucumber.

28. Lentils.

Lots of fiber and protein from plant

29. Mastic Perishables.

Minimal in carbs and versatile enough to fit into many culinary recipes.

30. Watermelon.

This fruit has a lower GI and is hydrating when consumed in moderation.

Remember to modify these choices according to individual dietary needs and tastes. Portion control and mindful eating are the two most crucial aspects of utilizing nutrition to treat diabetes. Consulting with medical doctors or registered dietitians may provide customized guidance based on individual health goals and requirements.

CHAPTER THREE.

Diabetes Friendly Recipes.
(Breakfast Recipes).

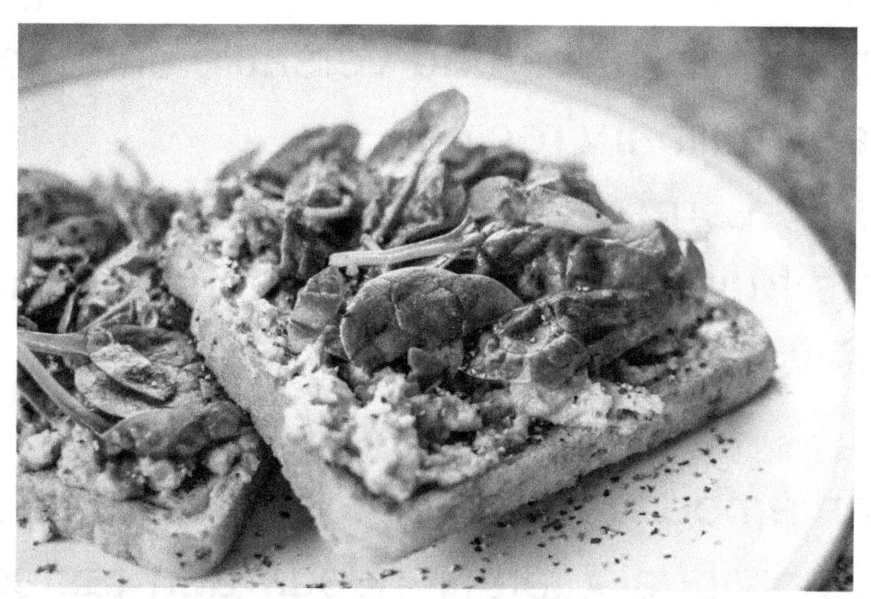

♦ FETA AND SPINACH OMELETTE

INGREDIENTS:

Using whatever unsalted or salted butter I happen to have in the fridge, I'll use two tablespoons of butter to make this omelet with spinach and feta cheese. But remember that feta is already rather salty, so use a little amount of salted butter if you use it!

• Dice one clove of garlic and one tablespoon of onion (I use whatever is available; red or white work nicely).

• Two large eggs, one-half tablespoon optional milk, one cup freshly cut and loosely packed spinach, two or three tablespoons finely crumbled feta cheese, and salt and pepper to taste

INSTRUCTIONS

Prepare your ingredients and preheat your pan for a few minutes before you start cooking.

Chop your onion and garlic into small pieces.

After rinsing and patting dry, cut your spinach. Beat your eggs (milk optional), and add freshly ground pepper to taste. I do not add any additional salt to the egg mixture at this point since the feta is already quite salty.

Once everything is prepared, put a pan over medium heat and melt approximately 1 tablespoon of butter. To ensure that the butter covers the whole surface and a little portion of the edges, tilt the pan gently back and forth.

Sauté the onion and garlic for two to three minutes, or until they become translucent.

Add the spinach and sauté until it wilts. Since spinach wilts rapidly, this should just take a minute or two to complete.

Remove the spinach, onion, and garlic from the pan; transfer to a dish and set aside. If there is a lot of liquid, you may layer the plate with paper towels to absorb it. I don't think this is usually essential.

Transfer the whisked egg mixture into the skillet, and if needed, add an additional tablespoon of butter. Depending on your pan and stove top, cook over medium-low heat for a few minutes or until the eggs are set.

Add the cooked spinach, onion, and garlic combination to the top omelet. Let the cheese warm through for a little while.

Once the omelet has been folded in half or thirds and most of the crumbled feta has been included, turn off the heat and allow the cheese to warm for a minute or two.

Spoon the remaining feta over the omelet after moving it to a tray. Considering that feta cheese has an extremely high salt content, season to taste with salt and pepper.

My favorite ways to serve my spinach and feta omelet are with a dab of good butter, some toasted crusty bread, and a fruit salad. Feta goes well with strawberries, stone fruits like nectarines, and melons like watermelon, cantaloupe, and honeydew.

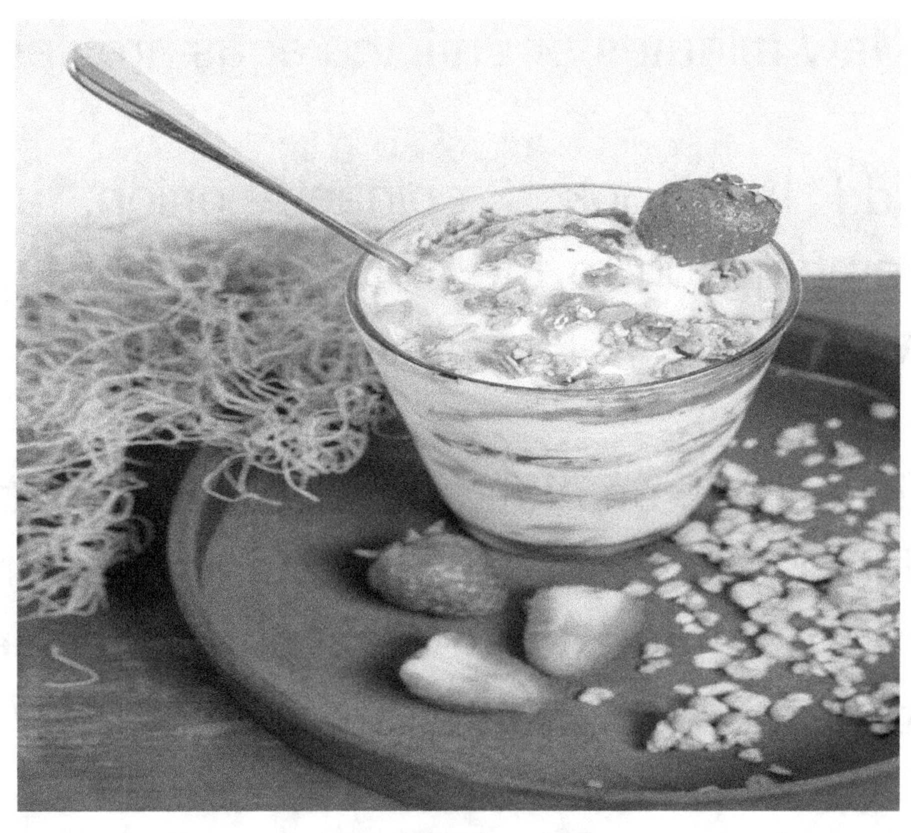

♦ GREEK YOGURT PARFAIT.

INGREDIENTS:

Any kind of yogurt will work, but I like whole milk plain yogurt since it has a thicker consistency and no extra sugar. I make my own vanilla Greek yogurt at home, but you could also use honey yogurt or even vegan substitutes like almond milk or coconut yogurt for this recipe.

Berries/Fruit: For this dish, you may use any of your favorite fruit combinations, such as my Breakfast Fruit Salad. I mixed up some fresh blueberries and strawberries. No fresh fruit at all? Utilize frozen fruit!

Granola: Call me biased, but I think homemade granola tastes better on yogurt parfaits and has less sugar in it than most store-bought varieties. However, store-bought will work in a pinch. If you're searching for a good granola recipe, don't hesitate to try my Chunky Granola. If you're in the mood for a high-protein yogurt breakfast, try my Quinoa Crunch for an extra serving of plant-based protein.

Optional Changes and Additions:
The coolest thing about it is making your own homemade parfait. These are some very good places to start.

Sweetener: Drizzle some honey, maple syrup, or agave over your homemade parfait as a natural sweetener. As an alternative, you might use my Honey Syrup, Blueberry Puree, or Fresh Raspberry Sauce to flavor the yogurt.

Protein Powder: Add a scoop of your favorite plant-based or whey protein powder to make a high-protein snack.

Superfoods: Include ½ teaspoon of hemp or chia seeds in each serving to up the nutritious content even more.

Nut Butters: Add a dollop of almond or peanut butter for healthy fats and protein. On the other hand, I suggest checking the labels for added sugars.

Nuts and Seeds: Are you trying to consume less carbohydrates? Take out the granola and replace it with a little handful of nuts and seeds. However, if you'd like a low-calorie yogurt parfait without any extra sweetness, feel free to omit the granola and almonds.

Chocolate Chips: Chocolate chips might be the perfect treat for you if you're craving something sweet.

How to Make a Parfait with Greek Yogurt

This yogurt and fruit parfait is really easy to prepare. To quickly cook a delicious and eye-catching breakfast, just follow these steps:

Add the sweetener (optional): Beat together your favorite yogurt and sweetener until the mixture is creamy and completely whipped.

Layer the yogurt parfait by spooning half of the yogurt into the bottom of tall glasses, bowls, or mason jars. Arrange a layer of half the fruit and half of the granola. Carefully spoon the remaining yogurt mixture into the glass, and then sprinkle the remaining oats and fruit over top.

Add the sweetener (optional): Beat together your favorite yogurt and sweetener until the mixture is creamy and completely whipped.

Layer the yogurt parfait by spooning half of the yogurt into the bottom of tall glasses, bowls, or mason jars. Arrange a layer of half the fruit and half of the granola. Carefully spoon the remaining yogurt mixture into the glass, and then sprinkle the remaining oats and fruit over top.

Garnish: If you'd like, you may sprinkle some granola, more fresh fruit, and a drizzle of honey or maple syrup on top. You may either serve it right now or put it in the fridge for later.

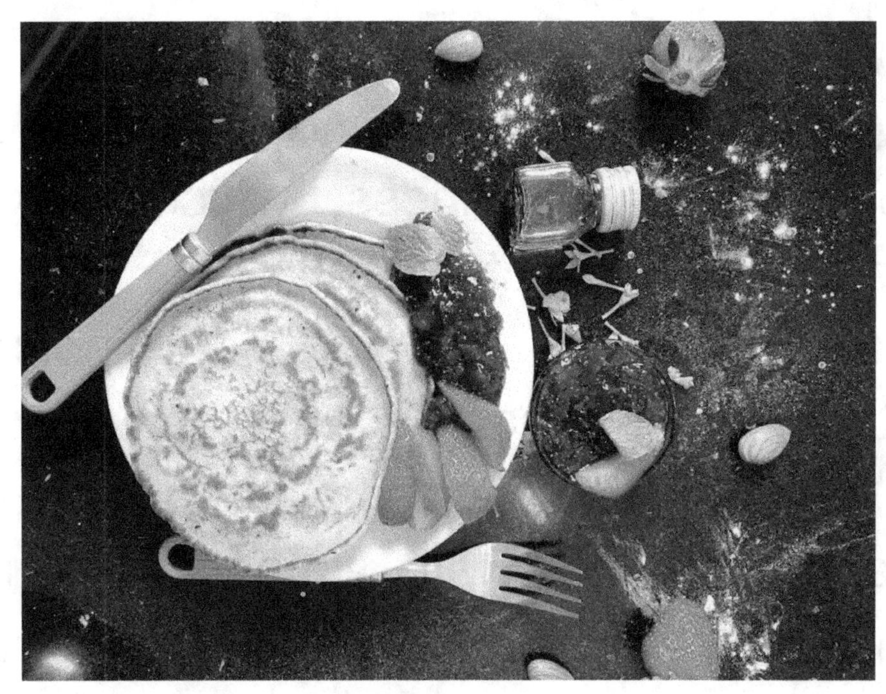

♦ PANCAKES WITH ALMOND FLOUR.

INGREDIENTS:

All you need for these easy almond flour pancakes are seven basic ingredients:

Naturally, almond flour! For best results, use blanched almond flour for this recipe or prepare your own using blanched slivered almonds. It adds to these pancakes' wonderfully light crumb and airy feel. They should not be consumed with almond meal since it will make them, well, mealy.

Eggs in the binder! They also contribute moisture and richness, which makes these pancakes very fluffy.

Baking powder: To aid in the puffing up of almond flour pancakes while cooking.

Almond milk: It adds moisture to this recipe for pancakes made with almond flour. If almond milk isn't easily accessible, you may alternatively use cow's milk or my own oat milk in this recipe.

Vanilla extract: It gives the pancakes a deliciously toasty taste.

Maple syrup: We will stir it into the pancake batter and, of course, drizzle more syrup on top when the pancakes are done.

And sea salt to enhance the hints of nutty sweetness and warmth!

Method for Making Pancakes using Almond Flour

Almond flour pancakes are a great alternative for both workday breakfasts and weekend brunches because of how simple they are to make. Here's how it functions:

Mix the liquid ingredients in a dish and the dry ones in a separate one.

Next, pour the wet ingredients into the dish with the dry ingredients and mix just until combined.

Now start preparing food! Heat a nonstick pan over medium-low heat and lightly coat it with olive oil (coconut oil would also be good). Using a 1/4-cup measuring cup, spoon the batter onto the pan; cook each pancake for 1 to 2 minutes on each side. Watch out for the color of the almond flour pancakes, since they will become yellow faster than regular pancakes. Reduce the heat if needed to keep the edges from burning before the centers are done cooking. Continue frying the remaining batter, and enjoy yourself!

Recipes for Serving Almond Flour Pancakes
The almond flour and eggs give these pancakes a robust texture, which makes them a filling meal on their own. Serve them simply or glammed up with Greek yogurt or coconut cream and your favorite fresh fruit. Even better, you could just serve them plain with a dollop of maple syrup.

They might be a great addition to a brunch menu for the weekend or a special occasion. I prefer to eat them with hearty meals like sunny-side-up eggs, my healthy breakfast casserole, or vegetarian frittata. After dinner, sip on a smoothie or some mimosas to wash it all down!

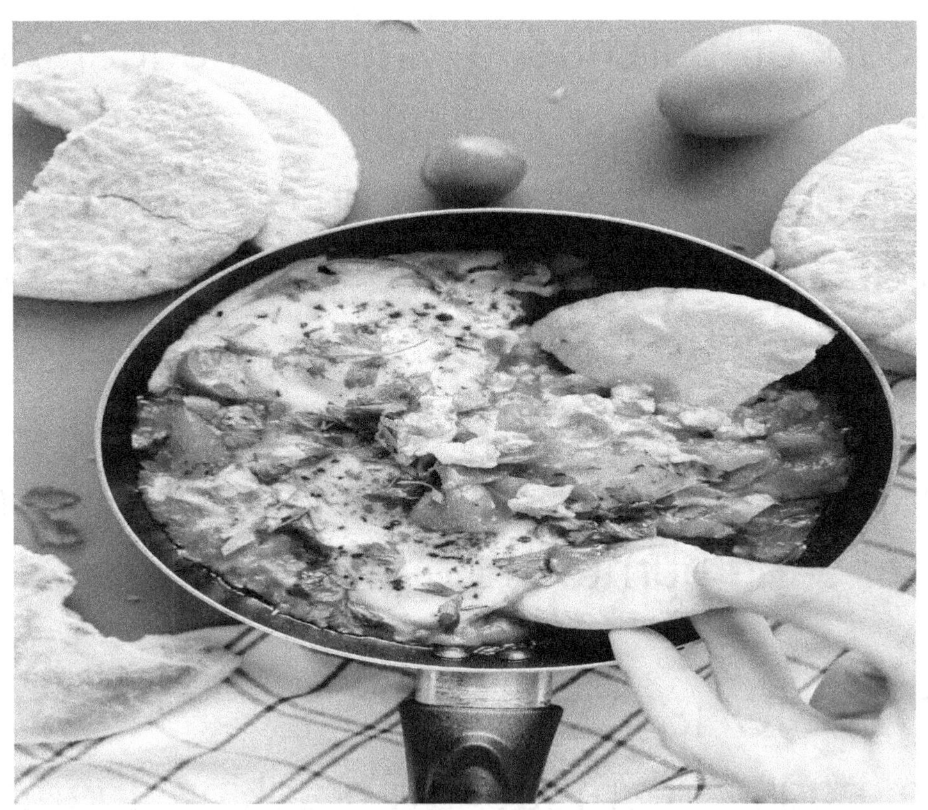

♦ VEGAN BREAKFAST BURRITO WITH EGG

INGREDIENTS:

Six 8-inch wholegrain tortillas.

A whole batch of home-cooked hash browns.

Six large eggs.

One cup of cooked black or pinto beans (I used canned beans that had been washed and drained).

Half a teaspoon of salt.

A couple spicy sauce shots, a la Cholula.

One tablespoon unsalted butter.

⅔ cup of purchased sharp cheddar cheese, shredded.

Chop up and divide a ½ cup of cilantro.

½ cup split finely chopped onion, mostly green.

Measure out 6 tablespoons of your favorite salsa and extra to serve.

Chopped one big avocado (not essential if serving the burritos right away).

DIRECTIONS:

The eggs are made by cracking them into a medium-sized dish and whisking them with a fork until they take on a light golden hue. Add the beans, then season with salt and the hot sauce.

Melt the butter in a medium-sized pan over medium heat (you may use nonstick or well-seasoned cast iron for this). This will cook the eggs. Add the egg mixture and cook, stirring often, until the eggs are just set, 2 to 4 minutes. Pour the mixture into a bowl after adding the cheese and stirring. Add the green onion and cilantro after that (if you're serving the burritos right away, keep a little amount of each for garnish).

To make sure each tortilla is beautiful and pliable, run it under running water for a few seconds (trust me). You may rapidly reheat the tortillas in the microwave or on a griddle (for 10 to 20 seconds).

Working with one hash brown at a time, spread approximately ⅓ cup of them about one-third from the edge of a tortilla. Drizzle one tablespoon of salsa over the hash browns. Scramble roughly ⅓ cup of eggs over the top. (Just be sure you divide the hash browns and scrambled eggs evenly; you may estimate how much to put on each tortilla.)

To partly wrap the burrito's contents, fold the tortilla in half from the bottom, and then fold in the two edges. After rolling, lay the burrito seam side down onto a platter. Continue with the remaining burritos.

You may serve the burritos whole or in half, as I did, if you're serving them right away. Reheat the burritos in the microwave or on the stove, then top with more salsa. Sprinkle the reserved green onion, cilantro, and diced avocado over top, if using. Use a fork and knife to serve right away.

Allow the burritos to cool to room temperature before wrapping each one in plastic wrap if freezing for a later time. Before putting the wrapped burritos in a freezer-safe bag, press out any remaining air. It is best to keep the burritos frozen. For best taste, consume your burritos within three to six months.

Once the plastic wrap is off, cover the frozen burritos in a moist paper towel. For two to three minutes, thoroughly reheat everything in the microwave. I like mine best served with extra salsa.

Notes:

Gluten-free: Make use of a tortilla that has undergone gluten-free verification.

Turn it out dairy: Substitute less than a tablespoon of olive oil for the butter and omit the cheese. Please provide avocado beside your burritos!

Make it quick: You may swap out the hash browns with an extra ½ cup of pinto beans.

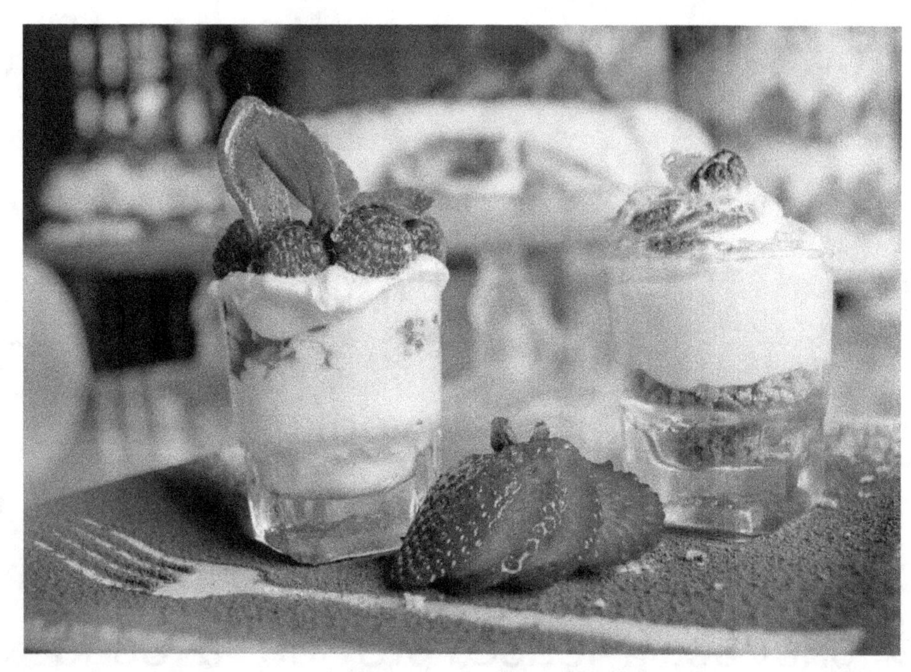

◆ PUDDING WITH CHIA SEEDS AND BERRIES

Why are chia seeds considered nutritious?

Chia seeds are a very potent ingredient. Just two tablespoons of chia seeds contain nine grams of fat, four grams of protein, and eleven grams of fiber (five of which are omega-3 fatty acids). Packed with antioxidants, they may help reduce chronic inflammation and support bone health. Chia seeds are definitely deserving of the term "superfood"!

INGREDIENTS:

Non-dairy milk: Almond or coconut milk are my favorites, but any dairy-free milk will do.

Any kind of chia seed ought to work! If you find that your current batch isn't absorbing as much liquid as you'd like, it may be time to buy fresh chia seeds!

I mixed blueberries, strawberries, and raspberries together to make my fruit. Either fresh or frozen works wonderfully for this dish! Other berries, including blueberries or blackberries, might potentially be used in their place.
A little bit of maple syrup provides a naturally occurring sweetness to complement the berries. Honey or agave are also effective.

Vanilla extract is another flavor enhancer that helps to balance the dish!

Two glasses of plant-based milk (my preference is coconut or almond).

Add half a cup + two teaspoons of chia seeds.
Half a cup of strawberries, either fresh or frozen.
A half-cup of blueberries, either frozen or fresh.
A half-cup of raspberries, either fresh or frozen.
Two to three tablespoons pure maple syrup, to taste.
One-half tsp vanilla extract

INSTRUCTIONS:

Step 1: Combine all ingredients in a large dish or mason jar and whisk. If combining in a large bowl is your preference, transfer the contents to a storage container with a tight-fitting cover.

Step 2: Place the chia seeds in the refrigerator for at least eight hours, preferably overnight, to enable them to absorb the liquid and flavor.

Step3: Enjoy it cold!

Recommendations for Storage

Chia pudding, if kept in an airtight container or mason jar, may be refrigerated for up to five days. You may dilute it with non-dairy milk if you'd like, since it will thicken over time.

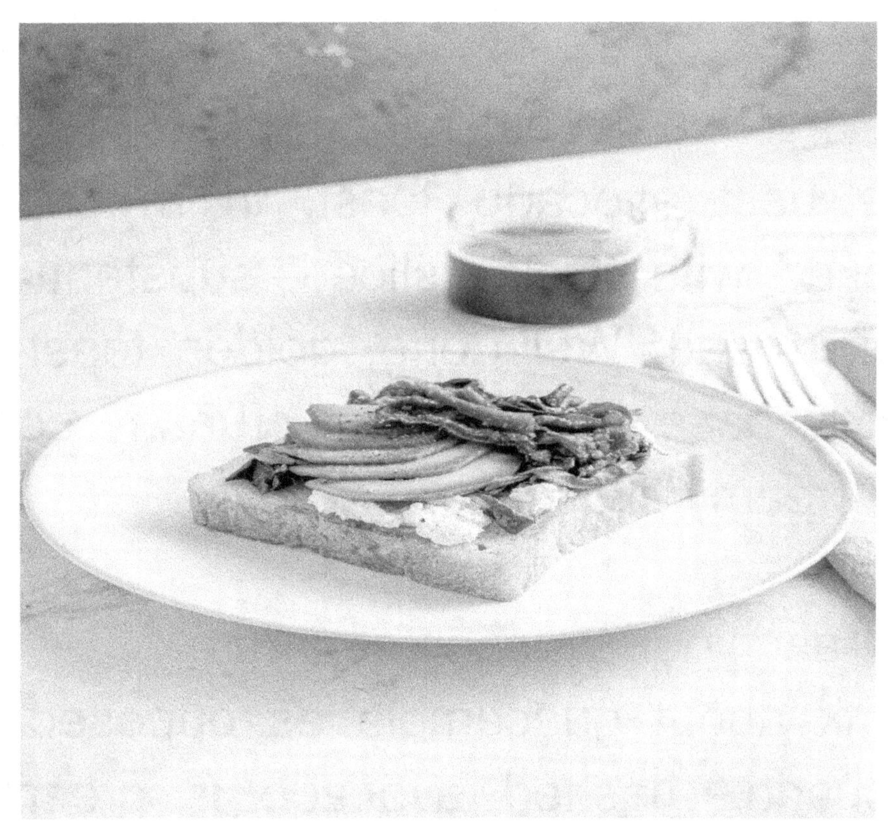

♦ TOAST WITH AVOCADO ON WHOLE GRAIN BREAD.

The Best Recipe for Avocado Toast
1) Pick out premium avocados.

Ripe but not overripe Hass avocados are what you desire. Select avocados that give slightly when gently pressed rather than ones with stringy or mushy interior. Before mashing the remaining pieces, remove any bruised or brown portions that you discover while cutting them open and discard them.

2) Purchase good bread and toast it evenly.
The best avocado toast, in my opinion, is cooked with thickly sliced, substantial, whole grain bread. Well-done, golden toast offers a sturdy base and a crisp, crunchy contrast to the creamy avocado.

3) Mash your avocado separately.
Think about guacamole as opposed to plain avocado; mashed avocado is creamier and more decadent than sliced avocado. But don't crush it on the bread! It's possible that you may pierce or shatter your toast. Cut your avocados in half, remove the pit, then scoop out the flesh

and mash it on the side of your dish or in a basin using a fork.

Mashing an abundance of avocados simultaneously? Instead of using that small little fork, use a potato smash or pastry cutter.

4) Don't forget to season.

Season each avocado half with as much salt as you can. Extra points? Toast with avocado and a little pinch of flaky sea salt on top.

Extra Advice on Avocado Toast

Here are a few easy and fast methods to make your avocado toast taste better. Choose one or more!

Add the garlic: Gently rub a peeled raw garlic clove over the top of the toast before adding the avocado, or mix in a little pinch of garlic powder.

Add your favorite herb sauce or some freshly chopped leafy greens (parsley, cilantro, dill, or basil are good combinations with avocado). Adding some chimichurri, pesto, or zhoug sauce—a hot sauce made with cilantro—is also recommended.

Add an egg: I like to top my avocado toast with a fried egg to increase the protein content (see here for an example). You may also create poached or scrambled eggs if you'd like.

Extra topping options include chopped cherry tomatoes, your favorite spicy sauce, or fast pickled radishes, onions, or jalapeños.

INGREDIENTS:

One slice of bread (I like my bread to be thick, whole-grain).

One ounce of ripe avocado.

A little salt, please.

It's optional to add any extra toppings that the bonus list suggests.

INSTRUCTIONS:

Toast your bread until it becomes brown and firm.

Remove the pit from the avocado. To remove the meat, use a large spoon. Move to a bowl and mash with a fork to get the right consistency. When necessary, add a little pinch (about ⅛ teaspoon) of salt and taste.

Avocado should be spread over toast. Enjoy the meal as is or add any of the garnishes suggested in this article (I personally recommend a little teaspoon of flaky sea salt, if you have some).

Notes.

To make it gluten-free, USE GLUTEN-FREE bread. My helper Megan buys the Canyon Bakehouse 7-Grain Bread from Natural Grocers, and it's a great bread.

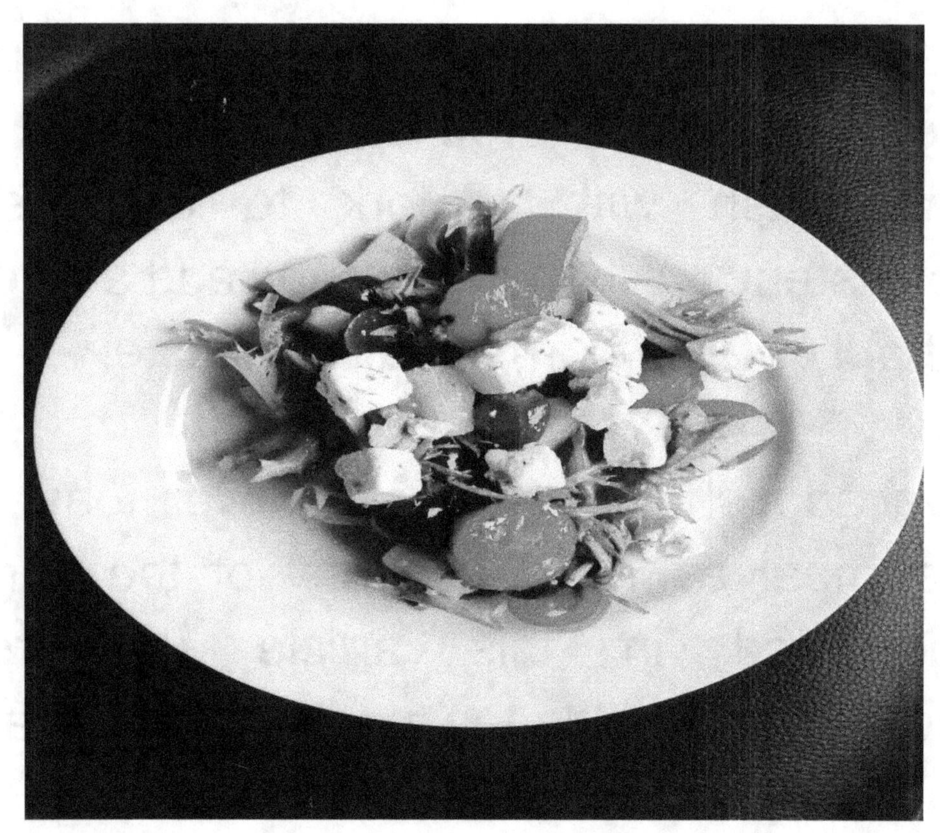

♦ PINEAPPLE AND COTTAGE CHEESE BOWL.

Why does this pineapple-cottage cheese combo work so well?

Flavors: The mix of pineapple and cottage cheese is very creamy, sweet, and delicious.

Simple to use, quick to prepare, and portable: This recipe only requires three basic ingredients and is very easy to create. There's no need for laborious cooking or preparation. Whether you're short on time, need a quick snack, or simply want to satisfy your sweet tooth, this recipe is simple to prepare.

Customization: Because this recipe is flexible, you may make it your own by adding or removing items to suit your tastes.

While the focus is on the mouthwatering taste, this substitute is actually rather wholesome. This kind of cheese offers calcium and protein, while pineapple provides vitamins and a delicious flavor all by itself. Honey is an optional addition for those who would like indulge a bit.

INGREDIENTS:

Cottage cheese: Select your favorite brand; it may be full-fat or low-fat, big or tiny curd cheese. You may whip it or leave it alone. You may use as much or as little as you'd like.

Pineapple: Use canned pineapple, ideally without sugar added, to keep the dish as health-conscious as possible. Pick the fresh pineapple that is the ripest and juiciest that you can find. However, if you use fresh, you should consume the combination immediately as it contains enzymes that cause dairy products to curdle and become somewhat bitter.

Honey: To add one more mouthwatering drizzle. You may replace it with maple syrup, brown sugar, or any other kind of sweetener.

We love cinnamon, but feel free to omit it. It delivers a burst of hot spices.

How can cottage cheese be made using pineapple?

Drain the pineapple well through a strainer to prepare it. Cut the pineapple chunks into bite-sized portions if they are too enormous. Before used, the pineapple should be completely drained. Pineapple crushed is also OK.

If the fruit is still fresh, peel and chop it first.

Use a blender or food processor to pulse the cheese (1,2).
Alternatively, take no action and let the cottage cheese stand by itself. We love its whipped creaminess, but real lumpy, curdy cheese tastes just as good; it all depends on your preference.

To flavor, add honey to dairy products.

To assemble, fill small plates or jars with a few slices of pineapple. Top with a dollop of cheese. Add the remaining fruit to the top.

Garnish with more honey and cinnamon, if you'd like. Alternatively, put everything in a large dish.

Additions and modifications:

Additions: You may also use other berries or chopped fruit. Incorporate some raw strawberries, blueberries, blackberries, or raspberries.

For crunch, add some chopped almonds or walnuts. This creates a delectable crunch. Shredded coconut may be used for texture and flavor.

Dairy substitutes: If you want a tangier taste, consider Greek yogurt for a novel touch.

Another alternative is to mix Greek yogurt with mascarpone or cream cheese, or even better, whipping ricotta. The dinner will be more appropriate for dessert as a result.

Spices: Add additional warming and soothing tastes. Give the pineapple a dash of cardamom, nutmeg, allspice, or pumpkin pie or carrot cake spice.

Add some fresh mint or lemon balm leaves as a garnish.

Make a smoothie: Process cottage cheese, pineapple, ice, and a little bit of honey to create a creamy, satisfying delight. If you use fresh pineapple, then have the smoothie immediately.

INSTRUCTIONS:

Fresh pineapple: A substance known as bromelain breaks down casein, the main protein in milk, when pineapple is mixed with dairy products. This procedure yields peptides, which are smaller casein fragments that are sometimes somewhat bitter.

Eliminate additional liquid: Use a fine-mesh sieve to squeeze out extra liquid if the cheese is too runny. This will help to keep the texture creamier.

Manage sweetness: Adjust the sweetness to your preferred level. You may add some brown sugar or a little amount of honey if you'd like it sweeter. To get the perfect balance, taste as you go.

In what way ought I to serve?

Serve from small dishes or jars.

Beat the cheese with the finely chopped pineapple and use the mixture to fill crepes or cover pancakes.

Pour more honey over the top and serve over waffles.
A portion of the mixture may be added to your granola, morning muesli, or overnight oats.
To make it a rich dessert, add more cool whip or whipped cream to the mixture.

♦ BREAKFAST BOWL QUINOA

INGREDIENTS:
A third cup of water, split

1/4 cup multicolored quinoa, washed

Two tsp of dehydrated goji berries or dried cranberries.

Just one little banana.

1/4 cup unsweetened almond milk.

A single tablespoon of maple syrup.

One-eighth teaspoon ground cinnamon.

Eight-second teaspoon of pure vanilla.

1/4 cup fresh or frozen blueberries, without added sugar.

One tablespoon of walnuts, finely chopped.

One tablespoon of finely chopped almonds.

One tablespoon of freshly picked pumpkin seeds.

Maple syrup and more unsweetened almond milk are optional.

INSTRUCTIONS:

1. In a little saucepan, bring half a cup of water to a boil. Add the quinoa as well. Simmer for 12 to 15 minutes, covered, over low heat, or until liquid is absorbed. After soaking the berries in

the leftover water for ten minutes, strain them. Halve a banana lengthwise. Halve a banana lengthwise and mash the other half.

2. After removing the heat source, fluff the quinoa with a fork. Mash the banana and stir in the almond milk, cinnamon, vanilla, and maple syrup. Transfer to another dish and stir in the banana slices, almonds, walnuts, pumpkin seeds, and goji berries. If desired, top with extra maple syrup and almond milk and serve.

♦ VEGETABLE AND SAUSAGE FRITTATA WITH TURKEY.

Prepare Ahead Turkey Sausage and Vegetable Frittata

This tasty vegetable frittata may be eaten as a quick and easy breakfast or as a wholesome, high-protein snack. Additionally, it satisfies the needs for macronutrients (high protein, low carb, low fat).

INGREDIENTS:

Blend of Vegetables
* 1/2 pound of ground turkey or chicken sausage (you can make your own; Italian or breakfast sausage is great)*
Chop one medium onion.
Eight ounces. sack filled with cut mushrooms.
One sweet bell pepper, chopped.
Cut a half cup of cherry or grape tomatoes in half, or slice and seed one Roma tomato.
Three to five ounces of recently chopped spinach or greens.
One cup of chopped roasted butternut squash or one medium sweet potato.
Mixture of Eggs
Twelve eggs (high-protein version; refer to notes)**

A quarter of a cup of milk (I like almond or cashew milk).

One teaspoon each of salt and black pepper.

Four ounces of optional cheese (feta, cheddar, or goat cheese work well in this recipe).

INSTRUCTIONS:

In a large skillet over medium heat, add the ground turkey or chicken sausage, chopped onion, chopped mushrooms, and chopped bell pepper. Break up the meat with a spoon and heat until it becomes no longer pink. Once the heat is off, add the chopped spinach or kale, along with the tomatoes, and cover to allow the greens wilt for 60 seconds.

While the meat and veggies are cooking, mix together 12 eggs, milk, pepper, and salt in a medium bowl.

Apply cooking spray to a 13-by-9-inch baking dish. Cover the chopped cooked sweet potato or butternut squash with the meat and vegetable combination and pour the beaten eggs over it. Sprinkle with cheese, if using.

Bake at 400 degrees for 25 to 30 minutes, or until the pan no longer jiggles when you gently raise it, and the center is set. Warm up and serve. I like to top with slices of avocado and salsa.

Store leftovers in the refrigerator in a sealed container for up to 2-4 days (or 4-5 days if you decide not to include the meat).

Notes

*All you need to do is add as many of the following spices as you have on hand to make 1/2 pound of ground turkey or chicken taste like sausage: 1 teaspoon dried parsley, 1/2 teaspoon salt, 1/2 teaspoon black pepper, 1/2 teaspoon crushed fennel seeds, 1/2 teaspoon paprika, and 1/2 teaspoon garlic powder, onion powder, and cloves.

Add 1 1/2 cups of egg whites for a higher protein version (more won't significantly change the taste). 1/6 of the pan's high-protein macros are as follows: 245 calories, 12 grams fat, 5 grams carbs, and 26 grams protein.

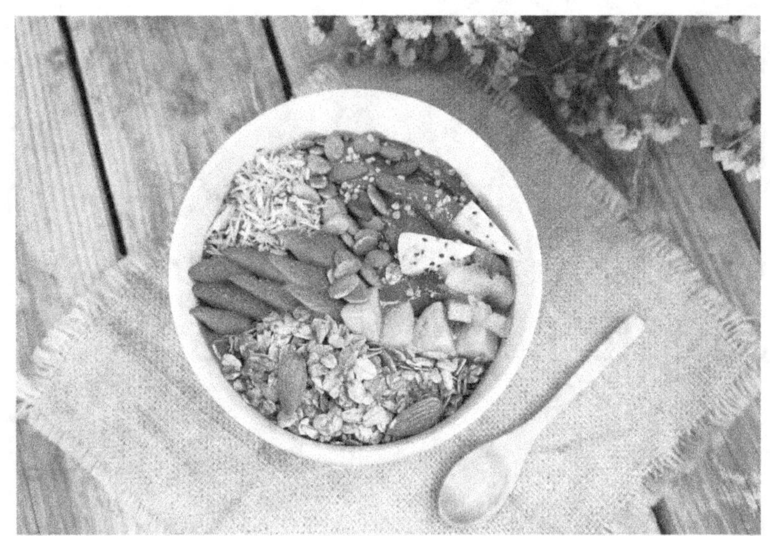

♦ WALNUT AND CINNAMON OAT CEREAL.

INGREDIENTS:
Take one apple, peel, core, and finely slice.
Three quarters of a tumbler of apple juice.
One-third cup of quick-cooking oatmeal.
One teaspoon of cinnamon powder.
One-half tsp of salt.

Two tablespoons of walnuts, chopped finely.
Two tsp honey.
One teaspoon of essenced vanilla.

INSTRUCTIONS:
In a saucepan, mix the apple, apple juice, oats, cinnamon, and salt.

Bring to a boil over medium heat and simmer, stirring regularly, for 1 minute.

Remove from the heat and stir in the honey, walnuts, and vanilla.

Cover and let it sit for five minutes.

♦ BERRIES AND SPINACH SMOOTHIE BOWL.

INGREDIENTS:
A single cup of frozen berry mixture.

Four ice cubes.

Splashes of light coconut milk (enough to get the blender going).

One spoonful of almond-based butter.

A little bunch of spinach.

Acai powder (one teaspoon) is optional.

PREPARATION:

Blend the frozen berries, ice cubes, almond butter, coconut milk, and spinach together in a blender. Add the acai powder while using it. Add more coconut milk if needed, then process until smooth. (As little as required to guarantee a dense smoothie). Taste and add your favorite sweetener or maple syrup if desired. Stir again.

Transfer into two bowls and top with hemp seeds, coconut flakes, dried strawberries, and blueberries.

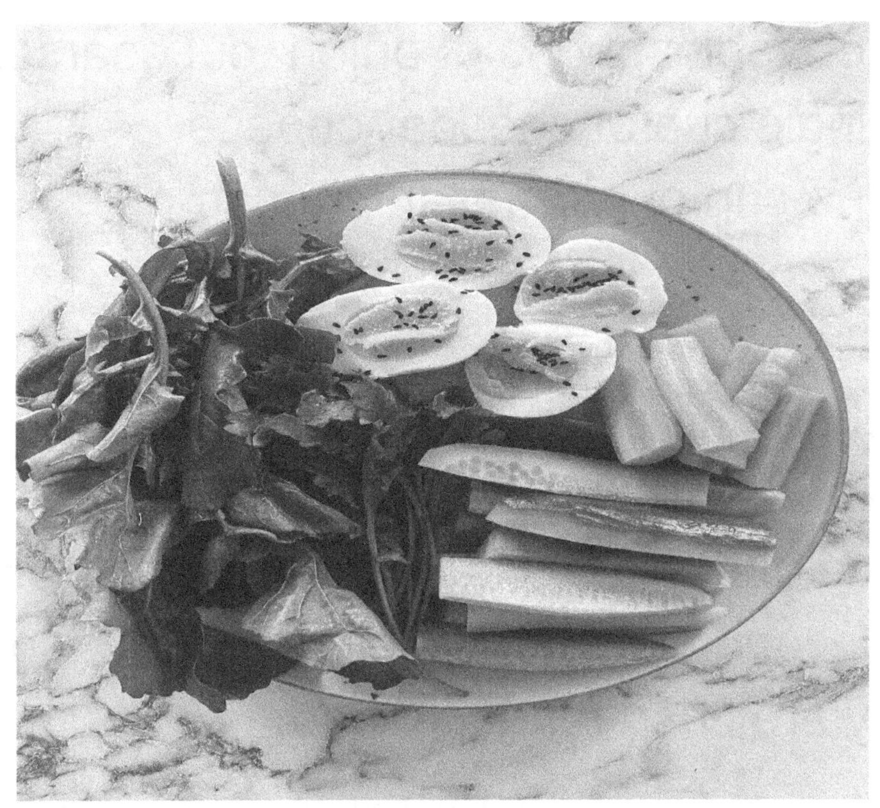

♦ BREAKFAST MUFFINS WITH EGGS AND VEGGIES.

INGREDIENTS:

Three cups of mixed vegetables, such as mushrooms, peppers, spinach, and broccoli.

A single tsp of oil.

A dozen big eggs.

A half-cup of milk.

One teaspoon each of black pepper and salt, or to taste.

One-half teaspoon of mustard powder.

Three tablespoons of onion, cut coarsely.
A single cup of cheddar cheese.
Half a cup of parmesan cheese.

INSTRUCTIONS:
Preheat the oven to 350°F.

Once the extra liquid has been drained out, chop and sauté the veggies in 1 tsp oil until they are crisp-tender. Good.

Coat a muffin tray completely with cooking spray.
Divide the vegetables, cheeses, and onions among the 12 wells.

In a large bowl, whisk together eggs, milk, and spices. Mix well.

Pour eggs into each well evenly. Bake until done, 22 to 25 minutes.

Remove from the cups and serve warm, or let cool completely before freezing or cooling down.

This tasty wrap with eggs and bacon is a terrific choice to grab before work or school since it has a whopping 27 grams of protein per serving! Prepare extras to freeze and pop one into the toaster oven for an easy and fast weeknight dinner prep.
High-Protein Burritos for Breakfast

INGREDIENTS:
Eight large eggs.
30 ml of 2% milk, two tsp.
15 ml or one tsp olive oil.

One teaspoon (15 ml) of coarsely minced garlic.

One red bell pepper, minced.

Half a minced red onion.

Four pieces of thickly cut, crispy bacon.

Add salt and pepper to taste.

Four flatbreads made using grains.

Fifty grams, or half a cup, of Mexican mix cheese, shredded.

INSTRUCTIONS:

Combine the milk and eggs with a spatula in a large basin. Set aside.

Put the garlic and olive oil in a medium pan and heat over medium-high.

When the onions begin to turn translucent, add the red pepper and onion and simmer for 3 to 5 minutes. Add the eggs, reduce the heat to medium, and simmer for a further three to five minutes, or until the eggs are set.

Place a piece of bacon and 1/4 of the egg mixture on top of each flatbread. Top with a little cheese. Enjoy it immediately or pack it firmly in plastic wrap or foil to go.

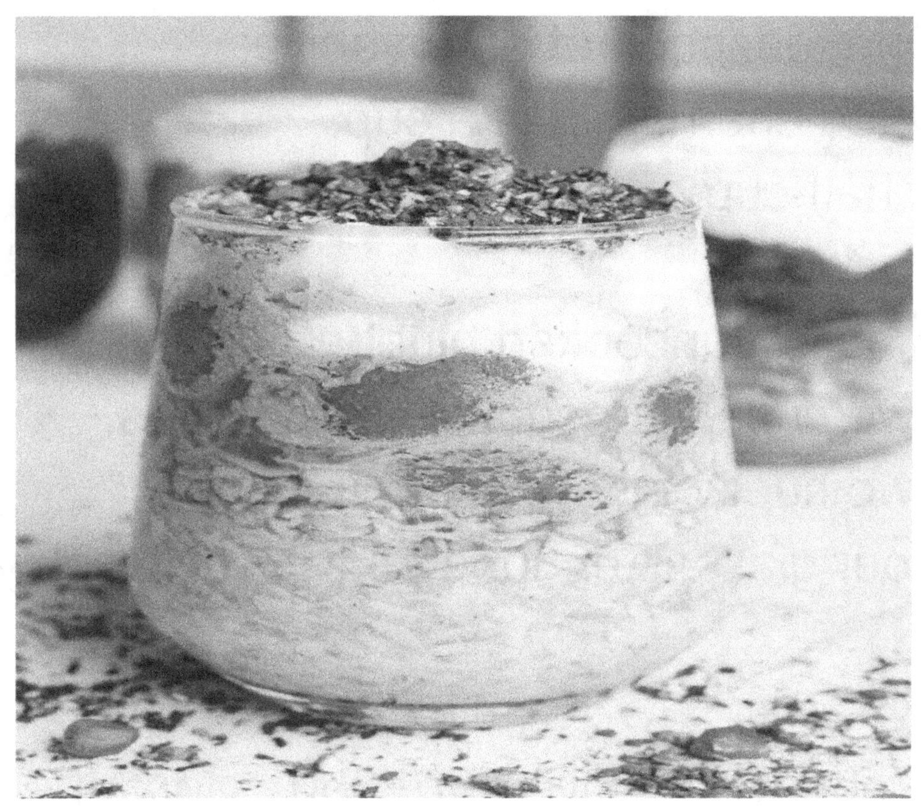

◆ BERRY AND YOGURT PARFAIT

INGREDIENTS:
A pair of standard oat cups.
Halves of pecans, half a cup.
Sliced almonds, half a cup.
1/4 cup of sunflower kernels.

Dense brown sugar, halved.

A half-teaspoon of salt.

1/4 cup of butter, cubed.

One-fourth cup honey.

One-half teaspoon of powdered cinnamon.

One teaspoon of pure vanilla.

Dried cherries, half a cup.

A half-cup of dried blueberries.

Parfaits.

A pair of uncooked blueberries.

Two cups of uncooked raspberries.

Two cups of just-cut strawberries.

Four glasses of honey-flavored Greek yogurt.

INSTRUCTIONS:

Preheat the oven to 350°. Mix the first six ingredients together in a large bowl. In a small saucepan, mix the butter, honey, and cinnamon. Cook over medium heat for 3–4 minutes, or until well combined. After turning off the heat, stir in the vanilla. Drizzle the oat mixture on top and toss to coat.

Transfer evenly onto a greased 15 x 10 x 1 inch baking pan. Bake until crisp and rich golden brown, 35 to 40 minutes, stirring every 10 minutes. Place on a wire cooling rack and let cool fully.

In a small dish, mix the berries. Divide the 1/4 cup of berries, yogurt, and granola among the 8 parfait glasses. Repeated layers are recommended. Top with the remaining berries.

CHAPTER FOUR.

Diabetes Friendly Recipes.
(Lunch Recipes)

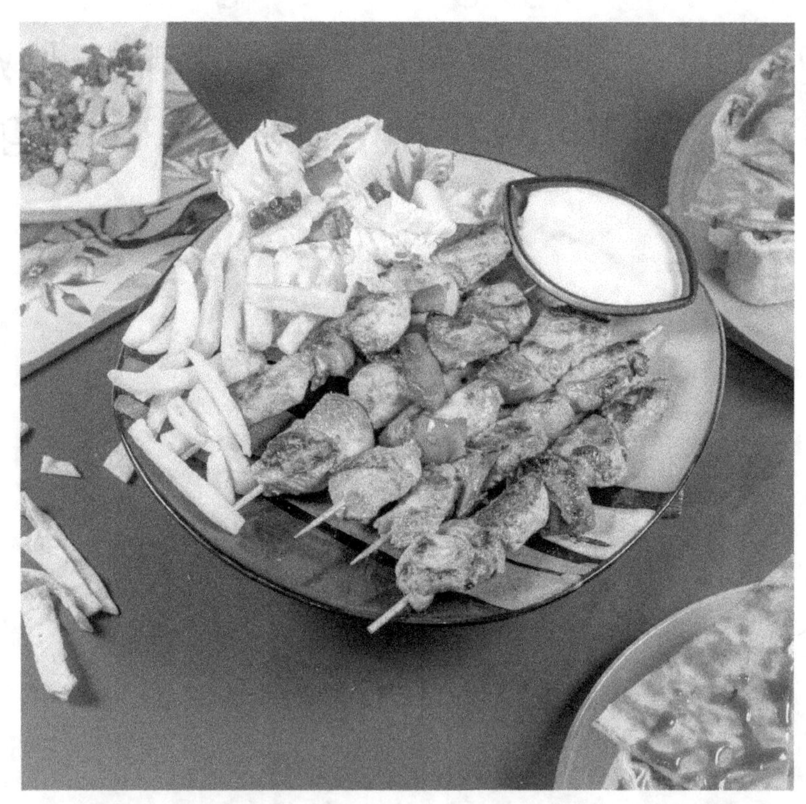

♦ SALAD OF GRILLED CHICKEN.

Grilled chicken salad makes an excellent lunch. It satisfies your appetite without leaving you feeling lethargic for the rest of the day since it provides you with a good amount of veggies and a modest bit of protein. We wanted to make sure you were satisfied with our version. That's why we topped this salad with some of our favorite toppings. This salad, which has avocado, tomato, feta, olives, and cucumbers, could end up becoming your new go-to work lunch choice.

If you don't have a grill, you may cook the chicken until the thermometer registers 75°C by placing it on a baking pan, rotating it halfway through. If you're a vegetarian or vegan, you may also use hard-boiled eggs or baked tofu. Here's a little suggestion as well if you want to bring this for lunch at work.

Rather than combining the dressing components separately, put them all in a jar or little Tupperware container. Just before you eat, give the jar a good shake to ensure that the vinaigrette is perfectly emulsified and suitable for a fine dining facility.

INGREDIENTS:

A pair of deboned and skinless chicken breasts.

1 teaspoon of ground cumin.

One teaspoon of oregano, dry.

Salt.

Ground black pepper that is fresh.

Extra virgin olive oil, five teaspoons.

One-fourth teaspoon red wine vinegar.

One tablespoon freshly chopped parsley

Four salads, chopped.

Thinly slice three Persian cucumbers.

200g of cherry or grape tomatoes, sliced in half.

Two avocados cut into slices.

Feta crumbles, 115g.

Kalamata olives, pitted, weighing half a kilogram.

INSTRUCTIONS:

Step 1. Turn the heat up to medium-high. To season the chicken, add coriander, oregano, salt, and pepper. Cook for 18 to 22 minutes, turning midway through, with a lid on, or until golden and no longer pink. Let it sit for five minutes before cutting.

Step 2. Meanwhile, prepare your attire. Mix the olive oil, red wine vinegar, and parsley in a small bowl and add salt and pepper to taste.

Step 3: Divide the lettuce, cucumbers, tomatoes, avocado, feta, and olives among four serving plates. Arrange the chicken slices on top and drizzle with the dressing.

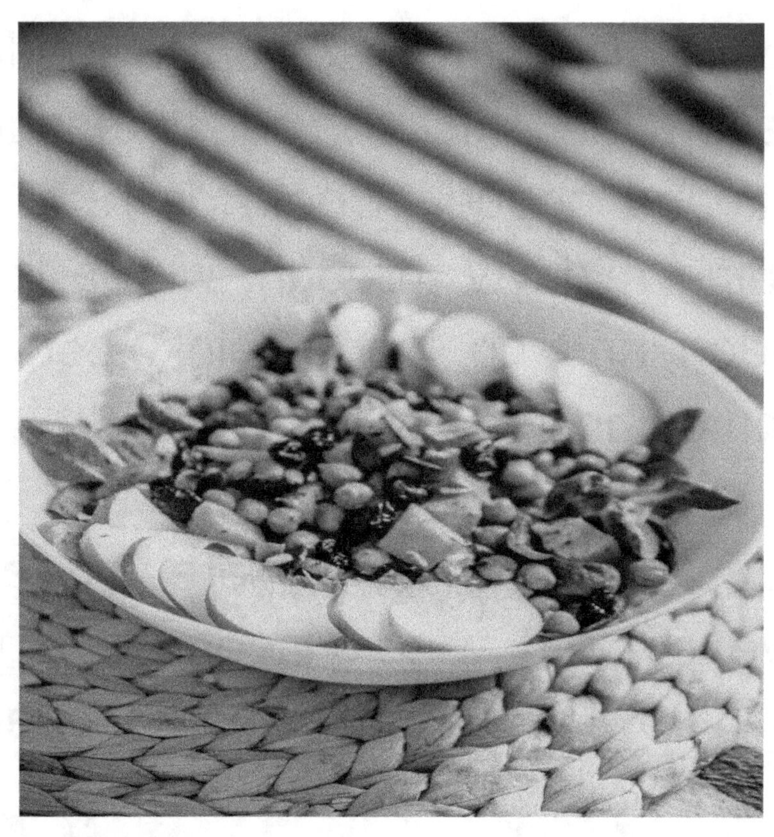

◆   MEDITERRANEAN   SALAD   WITH CHICKPEAS.

Whether we're craving something different and savory or simply can't bring ourselves to turn on the oven, we always come back to refreshing summer salads for our weekly dose. But occasionally, when we're desiring more than just a light side, we need to thicken things up, just like we do in our Mediterranean chickpea salad. Sorry, kale, but the chickpeas will fill you up for hours and make this salad really satisfying, but not in the way that leafy greens could.

The lentils are the main focus.

Canned beans are among our favorite pantry staples; they are really necessary. If you open, drain, and rinse a typical 15-oz can in thirty seconds, you could receive a one or two-ounce punch of real, reasonably priced nutrition. Regular cans are packed with of protein and fiber. Since you can eat them straight out of the can, this dish is ideal for summertime days when you can't resist turning on the heat.

This is referred to as a "chickpea salad," but you can certainly substitute any canned bean for the chickpeas. Excellent options include kidney beans, black beans, and creamy cannellini beans.

A shift.

Though we love this salad exactly as is, feel free to change any of the ingredients to anything you like. Do you dislike olives or bell peppers? Cherry tomatoes or diced ripe avocado might help to bridge the flavor difference. Would you rather not use dairy products? Swap out the feta for another protein-rich item, such as hard-boiled eggs, a handful of chopped toasted almonds, or a can of tuna.

Make it ahead of time.

If you cut all the veggies and prepare the chickpeas ahead of time, you may create this salad in advance and store it in the fridge for up to two days in separate sealed containers. You can also create your dressing ahead of time (we love to make extra to throw on all our favorite salads) and store it in the fridge in an airtight jar for up to 10 days. Before serving, simply stir everything together!

SALAD'S INGREDIENTS:

Cans of washed and drained (15-oz) chickpeas.

Thinly slice a red onion in half.

One medium-sized cucumber.

Just one bell pepper.

Chopped half a cup of Kalamata olives.

Half a cup of crumbled feta.

Kosher-certified salt.

Ground black pepper that is fresh.

Regarding the Violet Lemon-Parsley.

Extra virgin olive oil, half a cup.

1/4 cup of white vinegar.

One tsp lemon juice.

One tablespoon freshly chopped parsley.

1/4 tsp crushed red pepper.

Kosher salt.

Freshly ground pepper granules.

INSTRUCTIONS:

Step 1.In order to prepare the salad, place the bell pepper, cucumber, red onion, feta, olives, and chickpeas in a large bowl. For seasoning, add salt and pepper.

Step 2: Get the vinaigrette ready. Seal the jar and add the olive oil, vinegar, lemon juice, parsley, and red pepper flakes. Once the jar has been shaken to create an emulsified consistency, shut it and season with salt and pepper to taste.

Step 3: Toss salad with vinaigrette right before serving.

♦ THE QUINOA AND CHICKEN STUFFED PEPPERS.

INGREDIENTS:

A solitary spoonful of olive oil.

One medium onion, diced (one and a half cups).

Four cloves of finely chopped garlic.

¼ cup water and 1 cup of rinsed quinoa.

Three cups of cooked chicken breast, shredded.

One and a half cups of low-sodium marinara sauce.

⅓ cup of grated Parmesan cheese.

¾ cup of newly cut basil leaves, divided.

Four enormous red bell peppers, around eight ounces in weight each.

Two ounces (about half a cup) of shredded low-moisture, part-skim mozzarella cheese.

INSTRUCTIONS:

Step 1: Set the oven's temperature to 350 degrees. In a medium saucepan, the oil should be heated to a medium-high temperature. Add the onion and garlic, and boil, stirring occasionally, for 4 to 5 minutes, or until the onion becomes translucent. Stirring occasionally, add the quinoa and cook for 30 seconds. After adding the water, raise the heat to a vigorous boil. Cook for fifteen minutes over medium heat, covered. After turning off the heat, cover it and let it sit for five minutes. Stir in the chicken, marinara, half a cup of basil, and Parmesan.

Step 2: Remove the seeds and membranes from the peppers by cutting off the top 1/2 inch. Arrange the peppers cut-side up in an 8-inch-square glass baking dish. Cover it with plastic wrap and cook on high for three minutes. Remove the plastic wrap. Spoon 1 1/4 cups of the quinoa mixture evenly into each half of a pepper.

Step 3: Bake the stuffed peppers until they are soft, about 15 minutes. Evenly distribute the mozzarella. Once the cheese is melted, bake for an additional five to seven minutes. Divide the remaining 1/4 cup of basil evenly.

SUGGESTIONS: Bake the stuffed peppers until they are soft, about 15 minutes. Evenly distribute the mozzarella. Once the cheese is melted, bake for an additional five to seven minutes. Divide the remaining 1/4 cup of basil evenly.

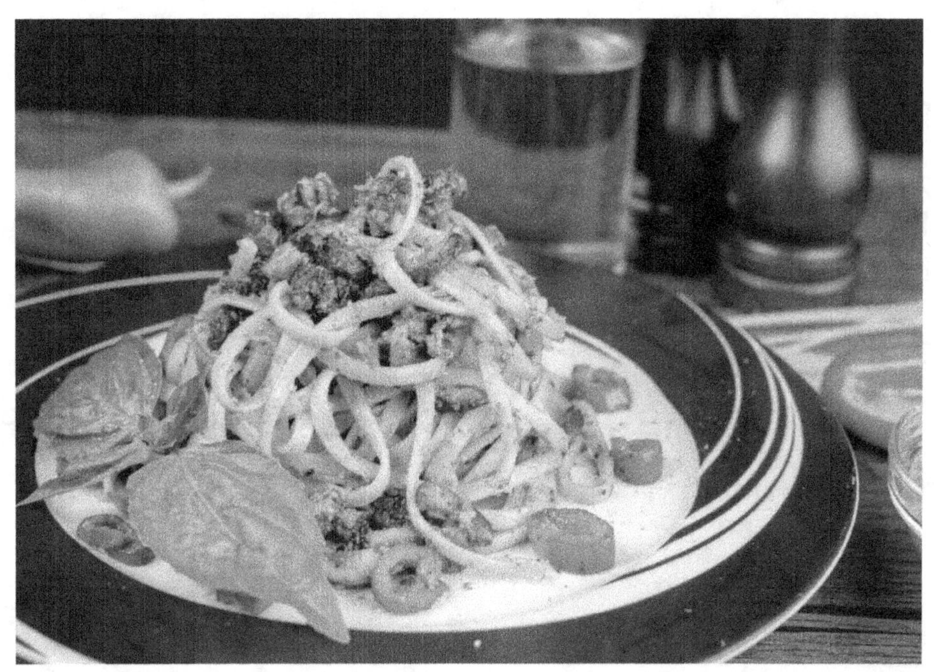

◆ PESTO WITH PUMPKIN SEEDS AND BASIL ON ZUCCHINI NOODLES.

INGREDIENTS:

Pesto made with pumpkin seeds and basil.

One little yellow onion and one clove of garlic, cut roughly.

A pair of cups filled with recently harvested basil leaves (arugula also works nicely).

½ cup pepitas, or green pumpkin seeds, toasted.

Olive oil, half a cup.

Two teaspoons of red wine vinegar, or to taste, lemon juice.

A pinch of red pepper flakes.

To taste, add salt.

Zest-based noodles.

Three enormous zucchini.

Salt.

A pint of cherry tomatoes fresh basil leaves for decorating.

INSTRUCTIONS:

To make the pesto, pulse together the olive oil, vinegar, red pepper flakes, garlic, basil, toasted pepitas, and onion (if using; see to the notes). After the mixture is smooth, taste and add salt (I usually use around ½ teaspoon). If the combination tastes too oniony at first, don't worry, it will soften in a few minutes. In an attempt to equalize the flavors, I added one teaspoon more vinegar.

To prepare the noodles: spiralize the zucchini using a julienne peeler, grate it lengthwise on a large box grater, or use a spiralizer to cut the zucchini into noodles (here is how to do it). Once the zucchini is well coated in pesto, taste and add salt (I used an extra ¼ tsp).

Transfer the cherry tomatoes to a large plate and spoon over the pesto noodles. Tuck the fresh basil into the corners as a garnish.

Observations:

*If you can't handle the taste of raw onions, avoid it.

*Toast the pepitas by transferring them to a medium pan and setting them over medium heat. Cook, stirring often, until the seeds release their scent and the pepitas start to pop, about 5 minutes.

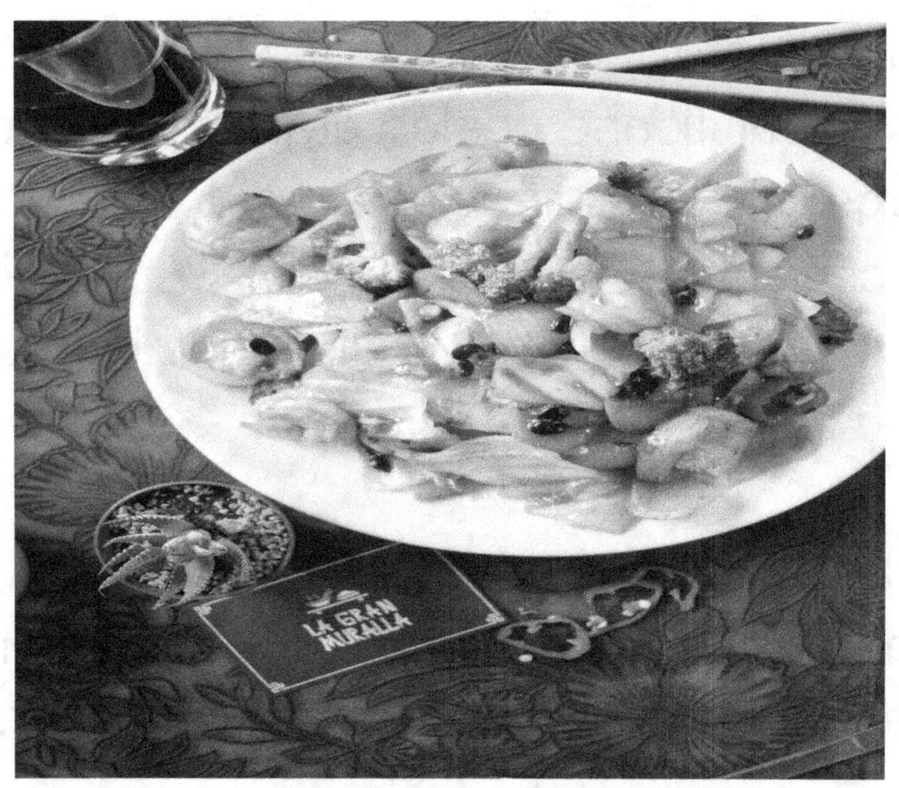

♦ STIR-FRIED SHRIMP WITH BROCCOLI.

This 20-minute stir fry is the easiest thing you will ever make, and it doesn't get much easier (or faster)! 287.3 kilocalories.

Stir-fries are among the greatest recipes. Because they are so versatile, you can pretty much use whatever leftover food you have in your refrigerator.

But I decided to make this stir fry really simple. Just shrimp and broccoli.

Because, believe it or not, these two make a marriage made in heaven. In less than twenty minutes, you can actually have this on the dinner table.

Just remember that cooking brown rice will take longer than the actual meal, so stock up on it!

Stir-fries are among the greatest recipes. Because they are so versatile, you can pretty much use whatever leftover food you have in your refrigerator.

But I decided to make this stir fry really simple. Just shrimp and broccoli.

Because, believe it or not, these two make a marriage made in heaven. In less than twenty minutes, you can actually have this on the dinner table.

Just remember that cooking brown rice will take longer than the actual meal, so stock up on it!

INGREDIENTS:

One tablespoon of olive oil.

A pound and a half of medium shrimp, peeled and deveined.

Twenty-four ounces of broccoli florets and one thinly sliced green onion.

A teaspoon of sesame seeds.

FOR THE SAUCE:

Three tablespoons of low-sodium soy sauce.

A couple of tablespoons of au poivre sauce.

One tablespoon of rice wine-based vinegar.

A single tablespoon of dense brown sugar.

One tablespoon of fresh ginger, coarsely chopped.

Two cloves of minced garlic.

One teaspoon of sesame oil.

One teaspoon cornflour.

One teaspoon of Sriracha is optional.

INSTRUCTIONS:

Combine soy sauce, oyster sauce, brown sugar, sesame oil, rice wine vinegar, ginger, garlic, and cornstarch in a small bowl. Stir in Sriracha, if using, and reserve.

Heat the olive oil in a big cast-iron pan over medium-high heat. Add the shrimp and simmer for 2 to 3 minutes, or until pink, tossing occasionally.

When the broccoli is done, add it and boil it for two to three minutes, stirring often.

Stir the soy sauce mixture in for one to two minutes, or until it is well combined and has thickened somewhat.

Serve immediately and garnish with sesame seeds and green onions, if desired.

♦ CURRY WITH EGGPLANT AND CHICKPEAS.

This flavor-packed, surprisingly easy-to-make vegan curry made with eggplant and chickpeas is full of spices. Forget about takeaway when you bring the tantalizing scents of your favorite Indian restaurant inside your home.

INGREDIENTS:

To make the spice combination, mix together the following ingredients (you may alternatively use your favorite curry paste or blend):

To taste, or one teaspoon of salt.
One-fourth teaspoon of coriander powder.
One-fourth teaspoon of ground cumin.
1⁄2 a teaspoon of the root.
If preferred, add ½ teaspoon of red pepper flakes.
1/2 of a teaspoon for cinnamon.
A third of a teaspoon of black pepper.
1/third teaspoon of cardamom powder.
For the chickpea curry, one large eggplant, peeled and diced (about five cups chopped), is required.

Twice as much olive oil as that.

Three cloves of minced garlic.

1 inch of ginger, grated.

One medium onion, cut coarsely.

One quarter cup tomato paste.

Wash and drain two 15.5-oz cans of chickpeas.

Two cups of water or vegetable broth.

One cup-sized bunch of fresh cilantro, finely chopped.

DIRECTIONS:

Add the salt and all the spices for the spice mix to a small bowl and swirl to blend. Set aside

Cover and preheat a 12-inch deep, nonstick skillet over medium heat. Add half of the chopped eggplant and simmer, stirring often, for about 7 minutes without adding any oil. To prevent the eggplant from sticking, you might need to add a few tablespoons of water at a time if you're not using a non-stick pan.

Place it in a basin after moving there. Continue with the other eggplant and add it to the bowl.

In the same skillet, heat the olive oil. Add the garlic and ginger and sauté over medium-high heat for about 2 minutes. Simmer the onion for five to six minutes, or until translucent, along with the spice combination.

Add the tomato paste and boil, stirring often, for three to four minutes. Add the drained chickpeas and cook for a further two to three minutes, stirring gently.

Add the cooked eggplant and the water or broth; cover and boil over low heat for 40 minutes before reducing it. Add the cilantro during the last ten minutes of boiling, setting aside a little amount for garnish.

A FEW TIME-SAVING TIPS:
Use any curry powder or paste you have from the store.

Use two skillets as opposed to one. One person will start frying the eggplant, while the other will start making the sauce.

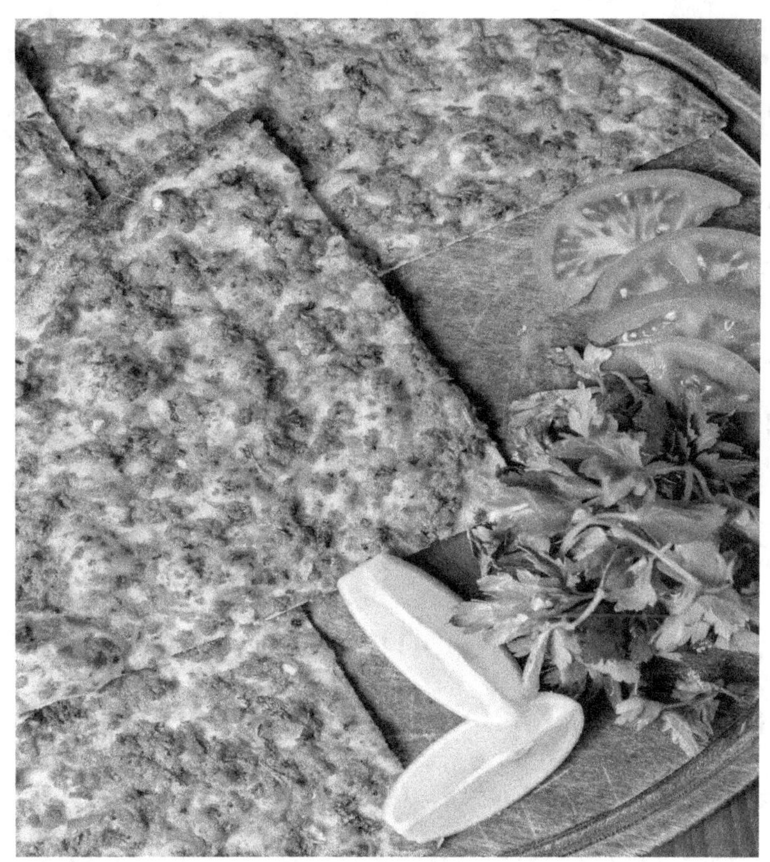

♦ PIZZA WITH CAULIFLOWER AND VEGETABLES ON TOP.

INGREDIENTS:

Cooking spray.
One-fourth of a large cauliflower head, cut into two cups of finely chopped stems and florets.
1/4 cup of Parmesan cheese, either shredded or grated.
Two large egg whites.
One large egg or a 1/4 cup substitute for eggs.
One teaspoon of dried oregano, minced coarsely.
One eight-oz tomato sauce can (sans salt).
1/4 cup roughly chopped fresh basil.
1/4 teaspoon salt.
1 1/4 cups of frozen, thawed crushed meat alternative.
Cut button mushrooms, about half a cup.
Half a cup of chopped orange bell peppers.
Half a cup of sliced yellow bell peppers.
Chop the green bell peppers into a half-cup size.
4 sun-dried tomatoes should be cut into 1/2-inch pieces.

Half a cup of shredded low-fat mozzarella cheese.

GLAZE INGREDIENTS:
Half a cup of vinegar with balsamic flavor.
A single teaspoon of honey Or one tablespoon of real maple syrup.

INSTRUCTIONS:
Give the slow cooker a thin mist of cooking spray. In a medium-sized bowl, combine the cauliflower, egg whites, oregano, Parmesan, and egg. Using your hands, press the ingredients into a crust on the slow cooker's bottom.

In the same medium-sized bowl (be sure to wash and disinfect it), combine the tomato sauce, basil, and salt. Spread over the cauliflower crust.

Place the bell peppers, mushrooms, and vegetarian crumbles on top of the tomato sauce. Sprinkle the sun-dried tomatoes over everything. Cover and simmer 4 to 5 hours on low or 2 to 2 1/2 hours on high, or until the mushrooms and bell peppers are tender.

Scatter the mozzarella cheese gently on top of the veggie topping. Put the slow cooker's lid back on and simmer for 30 minutes on low or 15 minutes on high, or until the mozzarella has melted.

While the mozzarella melts, combine the vinegar and honey in a small saucepan. Raise the heat to medium-high and simmer. Simmer over medium-low heat for 8 to 10 minutes, stirring occasionally and turning the pan, or until the mixture has reduced by half to about 1/4 cup.

Using a wide spatula, carefully remove the pizza from the slow cooker and place it on a work surface. Drizzle the pizza with the glaze. Cut the pie into slices.

How to Cook Sweet Potatoes with Stuffed Chickpea Spinach.

The recipe calls for my kind of multitasking with two distinct ingredients that go in the broiler right away.

The whole recipe seems really fruitful because the chickpeas and yams cook next to one another. That gives me a chance to focus on the spinach.

Usually, I sauté chopped spinach in a pan with a small amount of minced garlic, salt, and pepper until it has just started to dry out.

It is not time-consuming. It takes minutes to prepare the spinach.

When the potatoes are tender, I split them in half and use a fork to gently press the tissue together.

They can then be filled to capacity. I cook the fresh simmered chickpeas first, then the spinach.

I top these packed yams with red pepper chips and a generous dollop of tahini sauce.

These easy multitasking veggie-loving chickpea spinach packed yams are made by broiling all of the main ingredients at once in the broiler. Once finished, they are sprinkled with tahini.

INGREDIENTS:

Four sweetés.
Rinsed and drained canned chickpeas, 1–15 ounces.
One tablespoon of extra virgin olive oil.
One teaspoon of real salt.
Add another pinch of black pepper to the dish along with anything else.
One-half tsp cumin.
Typically, one cup of baby spinach is chopped.
1 garlic clove minced.
Twice as much tahini.
Sea salt, crumbly to serve.
Bits of crushed red pepper to serve.

INSTRUCTIONS:

Turn the broiler on to 375 degrees Fahrenheit. After puncturing the yams with a fork, cook them for 45 to 55 minutes, or until they are soft. Let the yams cool for five to ten minutes before cutting them lengthwise and using a fork to press their tissue.

Prepare the fresh chickpeas while the yams are boiling. Flush and channel the chickpeas. Use paper towels to clean them off. Remove any loose outer peels. Combine the chickpeas with 1/2 tablespoon olive oil, 1/2 teaspoon real salt, 1/4 teaspoon black pepper, and cumin in a small bowl. Arrange them in a single layer in a sheet container lined with parchment paper. Cook for 25 to 35 minutes, stirring occasionally, until the food is fresh and caramelized.

While the yams and chickpeas are cooking, place a large pan over medium-high heat and add the extra olive oil. Sauté the spinach for about two minutes, or until the passes start to shrink. Cook the garlic for another minute or two, or until fragrant, after adding the remaining salt and pepper.

Top each of the yam halves with spinach and chickpeas. Before serving, give it a quick tahini bath and a final dusting of flaky ocean salt and red pepper flakes.

♦ SALMON BOWL WITH TERIYAKI.
The Teriyaki Salmon Bowl is quite simple to put together. Over jasmine rice, top with avocado slices, sautéed spinach, carrots, and edamame, all covered in a homemade teriyaki sauce, serve heart-healthy fish (or chicken, if preferred). A few pieces of nori and a scattering of sesame seeds give it an additional kick of Asian flavor.

INGREDIENTS:
Two filets of salmon, preferably wild Alaskan king salmon, each weighing between four and six ounces.

About Teriyaki Sauce.
Soy sauce with two tablespoons of lower sodium content.

You may get two tablespoons of mirin sweet cooking rice vinegar (or dry sherry) from the Asian section of your grocer.

Two tablespoons sake or sherry.

Half a teaspoon of honey.

One-half teaspoon water.

One teaspoon cornflour.

FOR THE BOWL:

Jasmine is one cup of cooked rice, either brown or white.

One cup of thawed frozen spinach or two cups of fresh spinach.

One avocado, cut (½).

1/4 cup of fresh or frozen, thawed shelled edamame.

One carrot, grated.

One teaspoon of toasted sesame seeds, either white or black.

One thinly sliced sheet of nori, or toasted seaweed snack, measuring one inch in length and half an inch in width.

One green onion, divided into white and green pieces.

Preheat the oven to 400 degrees Fahrenheit. Put aluminum foil or parchment paper on a baking pan and set it aside.

In a small pan, combine the sake, honey, mirin, and soy sauce over medium heat. In a small bowl, stir together cornstarch and water while the mixture cooks. Add the cornstarch mixture to the soy sauce mixture and bring to a boil. Reduce heat and whisk regularly until the teriyaki reaches the desired thickness, which should take around two to three minutes.

Place the salmon filets, skin side down, onto the prepared baking sheet. Drizzle them with teriyaki sauce or brush it on. When it's done, save any leftover teriyaki sauce to drizzle over the bowl. Bake the salmon for 12 to 15 minutes, or until it starts to turn pink. Remember that once the salmon is removed from the oven, it will continue to cook for a few minutes. Let it cool for a few minutes. Take off and throw away the skin.

While the fish cooks, preheat a large pan over medium heat. When the spinach begins to wilt, add a small quantity of olive oil (or water) and sauté it for two to three minutes. Season with salt and pepper, to taste.

Before assembling the dishes, reheat the prepared rice and distribute it among them. Top with salmon, avocado, carrots, green onions, sesame seeds, edamame, and Nori strips. Drizzle any remaining teriyaki sauce over the meal, if you'd like.

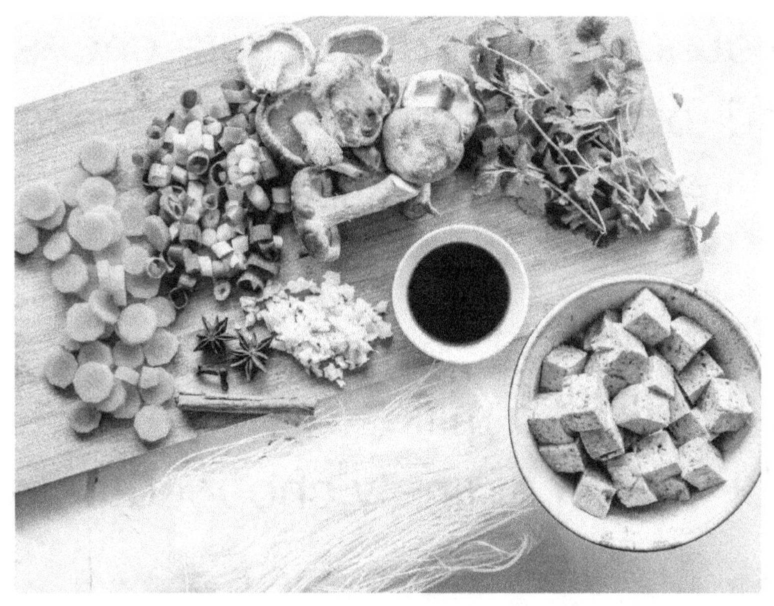

♦ QUICHE WITH SPINACH AND MUSHROOMS.

Perfect for any supper, this tasty vegetarian quiche has spinach and mushrooms. If you would like, you are welcome to add sausage. I usually freeze the leftovers after making two large pies or a huge number of small pies at once.

INGREDIENTS:

A half-ounce of uncooked spinach.
Eight ounces of freshly sliced mushrooms from one package.
½ yellow onion, cut.

Two ounces of crumbled feta cheese.
Shred four ounces of Swiss cheese.
One pie crust, ready made in a 9-inch deep dish.
Four large eggs.
One-fourth cup milk.
A tablespoon of finely chopped parsley, just now.
One teaspoon of garlic, cut coarsely.
Half a teaspoon of salt.
Half a teaspoon of ground black pepper.
One-half teaspoon of powdered nutmeg.

INSTRUCTIONS:

Step 1. Preheat the oven to 200 degrees Celsius, or 400 degrees Fahrenheit.

Step 2: Gently combine spinach, feta cheese, onion, and mushrooms in a bowl. Spoon mixture into prepared pie crust; top with half of the Swiss cheese.

Step 3. Beat eggs, milk, nutmeg, garlic, parsley, and salt and black pepper in a bowl. Pour egg mixture evenly over filling after swirling it around in the basin to distribute the spices evenly. After transferring the quiche to a baking pan, top it with the leftover Swiss cheese.

CHAPTER FIVE.

Diabetes Friendly Recipes.
(Dinner Recipes)

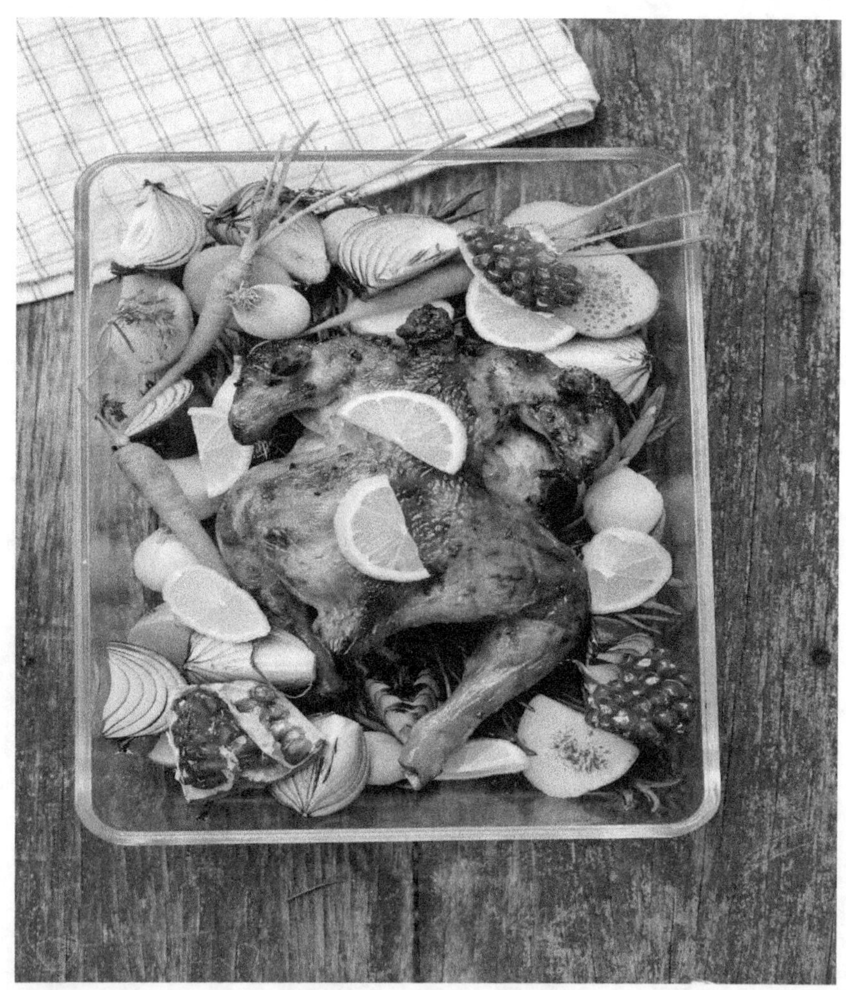

◆ GARLIC AND LEMON BAKED CHICKEN.

To guarantee that skinless, boneless chicken breasts are tender, tasty, and succulent, there are three essential tactics to follow. Learn how to make soft, juicy, and delicious roasted chicken breasts by reading on!

First, give it a marinade!
As per our recipe below, it's best to marinate chicken breasts for one to two hours before baking. Beyond that point, it is not required to continue.

I should mention that the marinade tastes well on all chicken and pork chops. Unquestionably a keeper!

The second secret is to cover the chicken lightly while it bakes.
Once the chicken has marinated, we gently wrap it in parchment paper (you may alternatively use aluminum foil). Loosely covered, the chicken breasts roast and braise at the same time. Because the chicken bakes

in its own juices, this keeps the breasts soft, juicy, and never dry!

Loosely cover the chicken.

The length of time the chicken breasts require to bake will depend on their size. Approximately twenty-five minutes in, we like to assess doneness and adjust as necessary. Most chicken breasts take around 35 to 40 minutes to bake.

Third Secret: Don't cook too much.
In this case, an internal thermometer is helpful. Bake the chicken breasts only until the internal temperature of the thermometer reaches 165 degrees. Any longer baking time will surely overdo it, leaving them dry and tasteless. Using a thermometer is the simplest way to ensure that the chicken is cooked to the right temperature.

INGREDIENTS:

It need two large lemons.

One tablespoon of extra virgin olive oil.

A single tablespoon of dijon mustard.

One-half teaspoon sea salt.

To taste, add up to 1/4 teaspoon additional red pepper flakes.

Half a teaspoon freshly ground pepper (black).

Three cloves of garlic, finely minced or mashed with a large knife.

A half-cup of recently chopped, loosely packed parsley.

Four 6 to 8 ounce skinless, boneless chicken breasts.

INSTRUCTIONS:

Give chicken a marinade.

1. After juicing one lemon to obtain 1/4 cup of fresh lemon juice, remove the thin, yellow skin by peeling or zesting it. If the first lemon's juice wasn't sufficient, use half of the second lemon to make the necessary 1/4 cup.

2. Whisk together lemon juice, olive oil, mustard, salt, red pepper flakes, and black pepper until the salt dissolves. Stir in the lemon zest, garlic, and parsley, if using. Use within 1 to 2 hours after storing in the refrigerator.

3. After adding the chicken breasts to the marinade, cover and chill for a minimum of one and a maximum of two hours.

GRILL THE CHICKEN

1. Position the oven rack in the middle of the oven and set the temperature to 400 degrees Fahrenheit. Coat a baking dish large enough to accommodate the chicken breasts arranged in a single layer. Grease the baking dish with one side of a large enough piece of parchment paper.

2.Halve the remaining lemon. Take off any large chunks of garlic that might have clung to the chicken breasts before putting them in the baking dish that has been prepared. After seasoning the chicken with salt and pepper, round it with lemon wedges, and place parchment paper over it with the oily side facing the bird. Over the chicken, loosely fold the parchment paper.

3. Bake the chicken until it is opaque throughout and the thickest part of the breast reaches an internal thermometer temperature of 165 degrees Fahrenheit. Proceed after around 25 minutes, after making sure the food is done. Most chicken breasts will require 35 to 40 minutes to prepare.

4. Let the chicken rest for about ten minutes, then slice it and return it to the baking dish with all of the cooking liquid (this is our preferred method).
Alternatively, you may serve it with some of the liquid still drizzling over it.

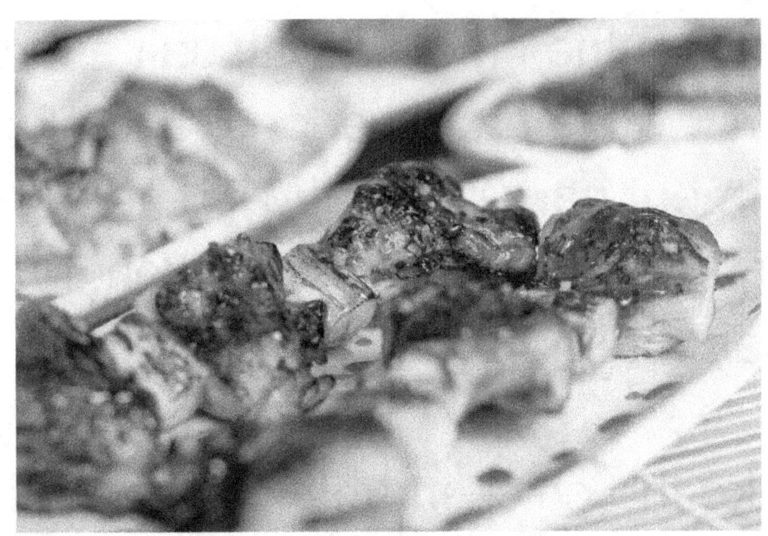

♦ VEGETABLE SKEWERS WITH TURKEY

INGREDIENTS:

Four hundred grams of turkey breasts.

A few zucchini.

Sixteen cherry tomatoes.

One finely minced garlic clove.

Four tsp olive oil.

Salted peppers.

Curry powder, two tablespoons.

1. Start by chopping the turkey into 3 cm (1 inch) pieces.

2. After cleaning and cutting the zucchini in half lengthwise, slice it into slices that are 1.5 cm (or around 1/2 inch) thick.

3. Thread the turkey, zucchini, and tomatoes in that sequence onto skewers.

4. Mix garlic, oil, and curry. Season the skewers by sprinkling them with salt and pepper. You can grill or pan-fry skewers. Cook until the meat is golden brown, about 5 minutes on each side.

♦ LEAN GROUND BEEF SERVED WITH EGGPLANT LASAGNA

This lasagna with pork and eggplant turned out to be a really tasty dish! These make delicious lasagna noodles, if you can locate them. Try ground lamb instead of ground beef for an additional variation.

INGREDIENTS::

Cooking oil spray.

Lasagna with nine noodles.

1/4 of a pound of beef mince.

One onion, chopped.

Four recently chopped mushrooms.

Crushed two cloves of garlic.

Two 14.5-oz Italian-flavored cans of crushed tomatoes.

Peeled and finely sliced one eggplant.

Two cups of mixed cheddar and mozzarella cheese.

INSTRUCTIONS:

Step 1. Adjust the oven's temperature to 175 degrees Celsius, or 350 degrees Fahrenheit.

Step 2: Grease the bottom and sides of a 9 x 13-inch baking dish.

Step 3: Bring a large saucepan of lightly salted water to a roaring boil. Once the lasagna noodles are soft but firm to the biting, boil them for ten minutes, then drain and leave aside.

Step 4: Cook and stir the ground beef, onion, mushrooms, and garlic in a pan over medium heat for approximately ten minutes, or until the meat is well browned.

Step 5: Add crushed tomatoes to the combination of ground beef and cook until a sauce develops, 3 to 4 minutes.

Step 6: Spoon about 1/4 of the sauce into the bottom of the baking dish. Noodles should be arranged over sauce. Noodles should be slightly coated in sauce.

Step 7: Cover the noodles and sauce with a layer of eggplant pieces. Arrange a quarter of the cheese over every eggplant piece.

Step 8: Bake in a preheated oven for about 40 minutes, or until the cheese is bubbling and browned on top.

Step 9: Bake in a preheated oven for about 40 minutes, or until the cheese is bubbling and browned on top.

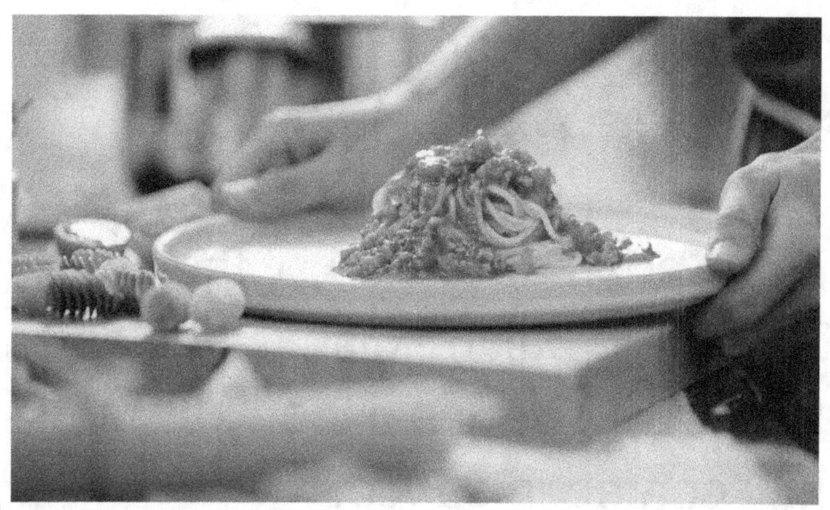

♦ ROASTED SPAGHETTI SQUASH WITH TURKEY BOLOGNESE

Roasted spaghetti squash with turkey Bolognese is a hearty Italian dish with a low-carb twist.

INGREDIENTS:

Three pounds of spaghetti squash.

Divide the olive oil by ¼ cup.

One pound of ground turkey.

Half a cup of 1/8-inch-diameter carrot dice.

Half a cup of yellow onion, cut finely.

One teaspoon of finely minced garlic.

Brown mushrooms, cut, in one cup.

Add three tablespoons of tomato paste.

28 ounces of canned crushed tomatoes.

One-fourth teaspoon dried oregano.

A teaspoon of kosher salt.

1/4 teaspoon of black pepper.

Half a cup of grated Parmesan cheese.

1/4 cup of Italian parsley, cut finely.

INSTRUCTIONS:

Set the oven temperature to 400°F (204°C) while centered the oven rack. Line a large baking sheet with foil.

After removing the seeds, cut the spaghetti squash into one-inch-wide rings and arrange them on a baking pan. Lightly coat the rings on both sides with a mixture of salt and olive oil.

Roast until tender, thirty to forty minutes. Use a fork to remove and separate the strands after a brief cooling period.

Heat two tablespoons of olive oil in a big, heavy skillet over medium-high heat.

Work the ground turkey into smaller pieces after adding it. While occasionally stirring, brown the meat for five to seven minutes. Transfer the cooked meat to a medium-sized bowl.

After lowering the heat to medium-low, drizzle 1 tablespoon of olive oil over the pan.

When the veggies begin to soften, add the onions and carrots, stir, and simmer for an additional 4 to 5 minutes. Add the garlic and cook for one minute. Add the mushrooms and simmer for two minutes. After adding, simmer for one minute with the tomato paste.

Add the crushed tomatoes, oregano, salt, and pepper along with the browned meat and mix well.

After lowering the heat to medium, simmer the sauce. Cover the pan, leaving only a little opening for steam to escape.

Simmer the sauce for at least 30 minutes to an hour, or until the meat is tender and the flavors have melded, stirring every 10 minutes. Add a bit extra water to the sauce if it seems too dry.

Over the roasted spaghetti squash, spread a layer of turkey bolognese sauce and top with grated Parmesan cheese and parsley.

♦ BAKED CASSEROLE WITH BLACK BEANS AND SWEET POTATOES

INGREDIENTS:

Chopped sweet potatoes totaling 2.5 cups.

A half-cup of cheese, shredded.

Salsa, half a cup.

One can of black beans, drained.

Shoepeg corn in one can.

Chopped 1/2 cup purple onion.

Take one spoonful of taco seasoning and use it.

One-half lime, squeezed.

Cut five taco shells into small squares.

INSTRUCTIONS:

Preheat the oven to 400 degrees Fahrenheit.

Using a knife, chop the sweet potatoes into bite-sized pieces.

Add the diced onion, lime juice, and taco spice to a large bowl.

Drain the beans and add them to the onions along with the corn.

Add the sweet potatoes and salsa to the bean mixture and stir.

And finally, cut the tortillas into little squares and add them to the bowl.

Spread oil in a 9 x 13 dish and top with the cheese shreds.

Bake for twenty-five minutes.

OBSERVATIONS:

*You may warm your sweet potatoes in the microwave for four to five minutes on high before adding them to the mixture if you want them extremely mushy. The recipe gives them a hint of crispness.

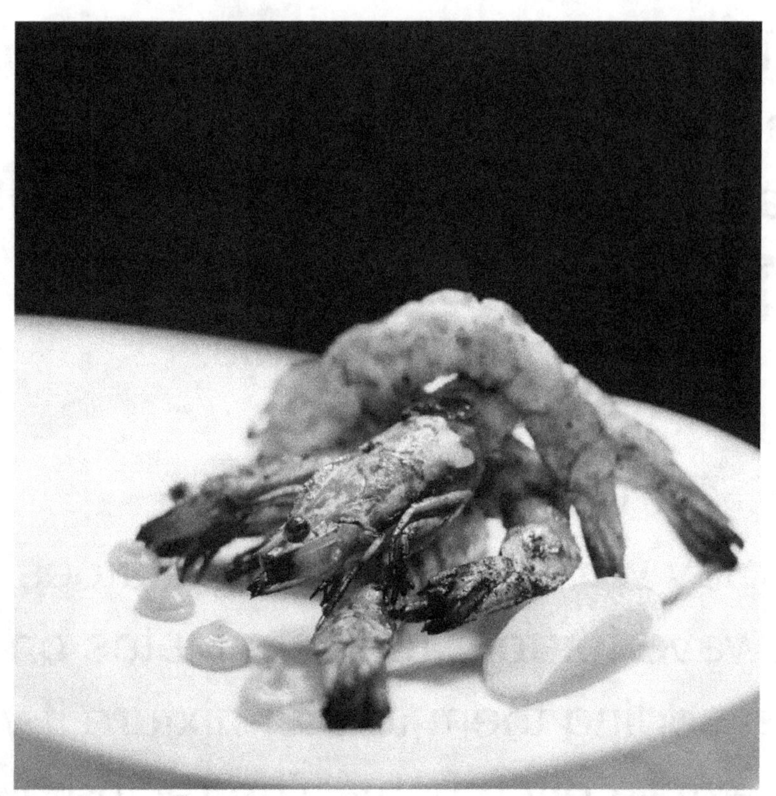

♦ SHRIMP WITH ASPARAGUS AND LEMON GARLIC

INGREDIENTS:

Four tablespoons of unsalted butter.

Half a teaspoon of crushed red pepper flakes (use less if you don't like spicy meals).

Four huge cloves of garlic, coarsely chopped.

1/4 cup of dry white wine.

Two tsp of recently extracted lemon juice.

Squeeze in half a teaspoon of fresh lemon juice.
A tsp of salt, or additional to taste.
One-fourth teaspoon finely powdered black pepper, or more to taste.
One-inch-long, chopped asparagus, one pound in quantity.
A one pound of defrosted, raw, patted shrimp.
A half-cup of freshly chopped basil (not too fine).

INSTRUCTIONS:
Melt butter in a large sauté pan over medium heat until just starting to brown.

When the garlic starts to smell aromatic, add the crushed red pepper flakes and sauté it for one minute.

Pour in the white wine, stir to incorporate, and reduce heat to a simmer. Add the lemon zest and juice, salt, and pepper, and simmer for two minutes.

Stirring occasionally, cook the asparagus for two minutes after adding it.

When the shrimp are cooked through, add them to the pan and simmer for an additional five to seven minutes. Stir in the basil after adding it.

Turn off the heat. Taste and adjust with extra spices or lemon juice if needed. Warm it up for serving.

♦ STIR-FRIED VEGETABLES AND QUINOA

INGREDIENTS:
White quinoa, raw, one cup.
One little onion, yellow or red.
One bell pepper—in my case, orange.
A pound and a half of mushrooms (I prefer cremini).

Ten ounces of asparagus, with the woody ends removed.

Snow peas or sugar snaps, six ounces.

*Omit if using an oil-free version. Two tsp toasted sesame oil.

Toss in some sesame seeds.

Regarding the garlic-infused stir-fried sauce.

A half-cup of soy sauce.

A third cup of vegetable-based broth.

Two cloves of garlic.

1 tablespoon of thickening agent, such as cornstarch.

Finely grated ginger, ½ teaspoon (optional).

INGREDIENTS:

Rinse and drain one cup of quinoa, then transfer it to a small saucepan with 1.5 cups of water or vegetable broth to cook. Increase heat to medium-high and gently boil. After that, simmer over medium-low heat, covered, for 15 to 20 minutes.

Meanwhile, finely slice the onion and bell pepper. Slice the mushrooms. Slice the asparagus into 1- to 2-inch sections after removing the woody ends.

Sesame oil* should be heated in a wok (or big skillet) over medium-high heat. When hot, gently add onions. Once added, simmer for three to four minutes.

Add the bell pepper, mushrooms, asparagus, and peas. When the food is crisp-tender, sauté it for six to seven minutes while stirring occasionally.

While the veggies are cooking, make the stir-fry sauce: In a small bowl, combine all the sauce ingredients, mince the garlic, and whisk to combine.

Reduce the heat to medium-low. Stir-fry sauce should be remade and added to the pan. To completely combine, stir thoroughly. Sauté for 2 to 3 minutes, stirring often, or until sauce thickens.

Fill bowls with saucy stir-fried veggies and cooked quinoa. Add more sesame seeds or tamari on top if you'd like.

NOTES.
* Option without oil:
Simply sauté the veggies in water or vegetable broth rather than sesame oil. (This works really well, but it provides a bit less taste.)

Vegetables: Change it up by using your preferred stir-fried veggies or seasonal vegetables. baby bok choy, broccoli, carrots, etc.

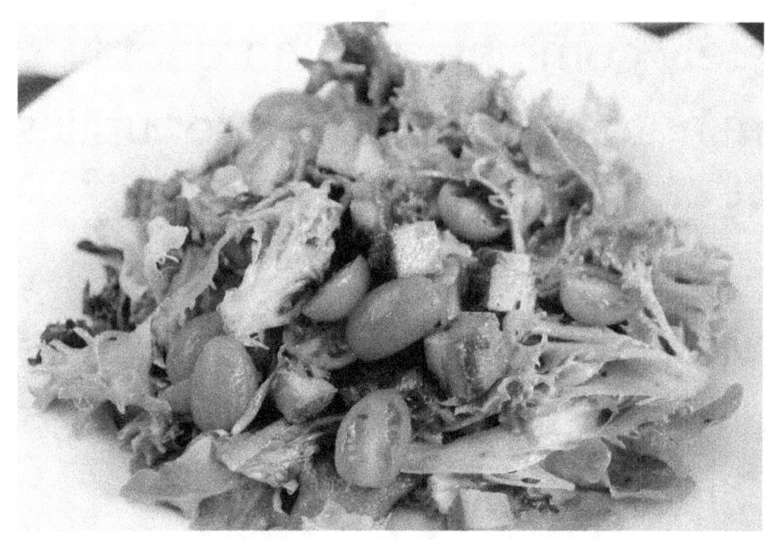

♦ GRILLED CHICKEN WITH A SALAD OF TOMATOES AND CHICKPEAS

INGREDIENTS:

US Customary Measured specifications.

A cup of uncooked barley.

One 12-oz filet of chicken.

Two tsp finely ground olive oil.

Cherry tomatoes, half a cup.

Two cups of cooked chickpeas.

Fresh bunch of sage.

Tsp of balsamic vinegar, three.

Salt and pepper.

INSTRUCTIONS:

Put the barley into a saucepan with salted water and heat it to a boiling point. After it comes to a boil, lower the heat, cover, and simmer for approximately 30 minutes or until it becomes soft. Drain, rinse, and set aside.

On a heated griddle, grill the chicken over medium-high heat for two minutes on each side (more if the cut is thicker). Once cooked, chop them and set them aside.

In a skillet over medium heat, add the extra virgin olive oil and sauté the tomatoes for one minute.

Add the chickpeas, barley, and sage and stir. Toss for five minutes.

Add the chicken as well.

For seasoning, add the balsamic vinegar, salt, and pepper. Throw for a minute.

Reheat and proceed to serve.

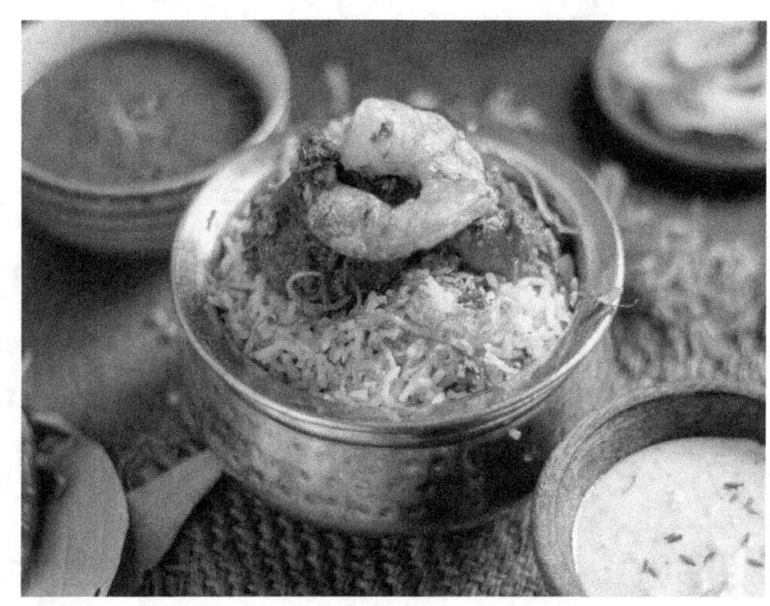

♦ SHRIMP AND CAULIFLOWER FRIED RICE

Regarding the Shrimp.
One pound of shrimp, deveined, skinned, and tail removed.
Add salt and pepper to taste.
Twice as much olive oil as that.
1/4 tspn oil of roasted sesame.
About the "Rice" that is Fried.
One cup of diced carrot, or about one carrot.
Half an onion or one cup of chopped onion.

Two cloves of minced garlic.

Half a head, or two cups, of broccoli florets.

Twice as much olive oil as that.

One teaspoon of toasted sesame oil.

A pair of eggs.

Cauliflower rice in two cups.

Three thinly sliced scallions (only the green or light green section).

One-fourth teaspoon of sesame seeds, toasted.

Coconut amino acids, one tablespoon.

To taste, add red pepper flakes (optional).

Add salt and pepper to taste.

INSTRUCTIONS:

Heat the olive and sesame oils in a large pan over medium-high heat. For three minutes, sauté the onions, carrots, and garlic. Season with a touch of salt and pepper.

Add the broccoli florets and sauté, stirring occasionally, for an additional five minutes.

Meanwhile, cook the shrimp by heating up 1 tablespoon olive oil and 1/2 teaspoon sesame oil over medium-high heat. To make sure the oil coats the bottom of the pan uniformly, stir the pan. Sear the shrimp for 3–4 minutes on each side, or until the edges are gently brown and the shrimp are cooked through. Switch off the heat and set aside so that the "rice" has time to complete.

While the veggies are sautéing, lower the heat to medium-low. Empty one side of the pan after moving all the veggies to the other. Whisk the two eggs together in a small dish and pour onto the uncovered side of the pan. Allow them to settle for about two minutes, then scramble them until cooked through.

Add the riced cauliflower and scallions and continue to sauté until the cauliflower is soft and cooked through, about 3 more minutes.

Add the coconut aminos, crushed red pepper, and salt and pepper to taste, if needed.

Add the cooked shrimp and mix once more. Sprinkle some toasted sesame seeds on top.

Be present and relish!

♦ QUINOA TABBOULEH WITH BAKED LEMON COD

Our whole grain-based lemon cod dish tastes great and is reduced in oil, saturated fat, and salt. You may use bulgar wheat or couscous in place of the quinoa if you'd like something a bit different. Delectable.

INGREDIENTS:

A 200-gram quinoa.
Zest and juice one lemon.
Four tomatoes, chopped.
Parsley, chopped, in a 25g container.
Four 200g filets of cod.
Hemp oil, cold-pressed, two teaspoons.

How to Bake Quinoa Tabbouleh with Lemon Cod:

To begin with, preheat the oven to 200°C, or gas mark 6.

Cook the quinoa in boiling water for 15 minutes, then drain and cool in cold water to make the tabbouleh. Stir in the tomato, parsley, and lemon juice. For taste, add a small pinch of black pepper.

In the meanwhile, place the fish on a lightly greased baking pan. Drizzle the fish with a black pepper-seasoned combination of lemon zest and rapeseed oil. Bake until heated through, 15 to 20 minutes.

Arrange the fish on top of the quinoa-based tabbouleh.

Recipe Advice:
Instead of using quinoa, think about substituting bulgur wheat or couscous.

CHAPTER SIX.

Diabetes Friendly Recipes.
(Smoothie Recipes)

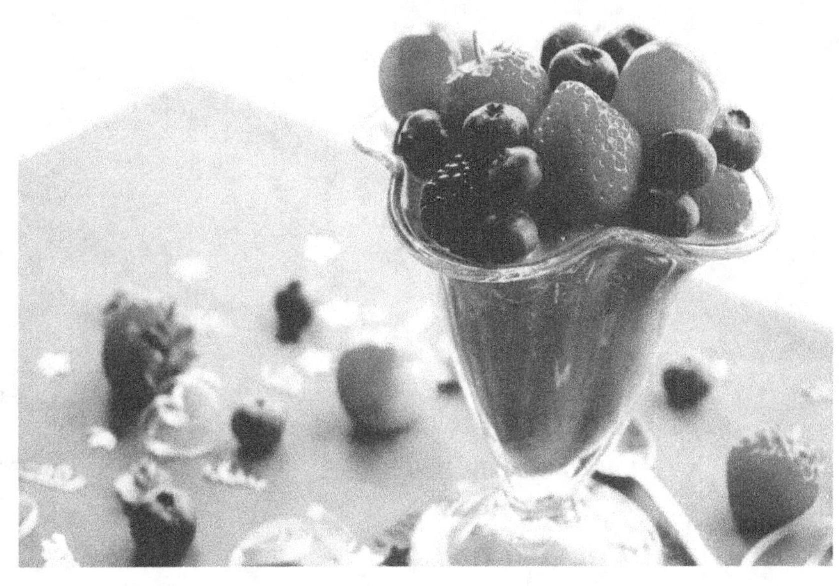

♦ SMOOTHIE BERRY BLAST

INGREDIENTS:

One cup of blueberries, raspberries, and strawberries combined.
1½ cups of yogurt.

A half-cup of milk.
One tablespoon honey, or any other sweetener
of your choice (optional).
Ice cubes (optional, for a cooler smoothie).

INSTRUCTIONS:
Assemble each element:

Remove any stems or leaves from the berries
after giving them a thorough rinsing.

In a blender, combine the yogurt, milk, honey,
and other berries, if desired.

If you want your smoothie to be cooler, add
some ice cubes to the blender.

Process the components quickly until a smooth
and well-combined mixture is achieved.

Taste the smoothie and adjust the sweetness
with extra honey or sweetener if needed.

Pour the Berry Blast Smoothie into cups and serve immediately.

*A Recipe for the Perfect Smoothie.
For a creamier smoothie, use frozen fruit or stir in a dollop of Greek yogurt. To make it sweeter, try adding agave nectar or honey, which are natural sweeteners.

Health Benefits of the Berry Blast Smoothie: Berries are a great source of antioxidants, which help the body fight off free radicals. Additionally, they are high in fiber, which is beneficial to the digestive system. Because it has protein from the milk or yogurt to help keep you satisfied, this smoothie is a terrific choice for a quick breakfast or snack.

♦ SMOOTHIE TROPICAL PARADISE

INGREDIENTS:

Before we begin, let's gather all the ingredients for our Tropical Paradise Smoothie:

One banana that is ripe.

Frozen pineapple chunks, one cup.

Frozen mango chunks, one cup.

A single cup of coconut water.

Almond milk in a cup.

A single spoonful of honey.

Chia seeds, one tablespoon.

INSTRUCTIONS:

Now that everything is ready, let's make this delicious smoothie by following the instructions:

Step 1: Gather each element. Make sure you have all of the items stated above before you start.

Step 2: Chop the fully grown banana and peel it. This will help the smoothie incorporate the banana more smoothly.

Step 3: Add the frozen pineapple pieces to the blender. The frozen pineapple will give the smoothie a wonderful texture and a hint of tropical taste.

Step 4: Add the frozen mango pieces to the blender. The pineapple will complement the frozen mango's creamy, tart taste in the smoothie.

Step 5: Include the coconut water and almond milk. These liquids will give the smoothie a smooth smoothness and a bit of nutty taste from the almond milk.

Step 6: Add the banana slices to the blender. Because of the ripe banana, the smoothie will naturally be sweet and creamy.

Step 7: Drizzle a little honey over the ingredients. The natural sweetness of the fruits will be enhanced and given a hint of sweetness by honey.

Step 8: Add the chia seeds as a garnish. Chia seeds are an excellent source of fiber and will provide a subtle crunch to the smoothie.

Step 9: Blend everything together until smooth and creamy. Process everything at a high speed until all the ingredients are fully blended and the smoothie is smooth and creamy.

Step 10: Pour into glasses and serve right away. Enjoy this tropical paradise smoothie fresh for optimum taste and refreshing delight.

The benefits of the tropical paradise smoothie
Not only is this Tropical Paradise Smoothie delicious and refreshing, but it also has a lot of health benefits. Let's look at a few benefits that this smoothie offers:

Delicious Taste: The way the mango, pineapple, and juicy banana come together to produce a flavor explosion in your mouth makes this smoothie a real pleasure to appreciate.

Hydration: This smoothie is a terrific way to remain hydrated, especially on hot summer days. It contains hydrating ingredients like almond milk and coconut water.

Nutritious Value: Packed with vitamins, minerals, and antioxidants from the tropical fruits, this smoothie is a terrific way to get additional nutrition into your diet.

Boosts Immune System: The high vitamin C content of the fruits aids in strengthening and illness prevention of your immune system.

Promotes Digestive Health: The fiber in the chia seeds and fruits aids in digestion and keeps your digestive system functioning well.

Gives Energy: The natural sugars in the fruits plus the ingredients' capacity to provide a quick energy boost make this smoothie a fantastic choice for a midday pick-me-up.

Supports Weight reduction: The fiber and low calorie content of this smoothie will help you reach your weight reduction goals by making you feel satisfied for longer.

Rich in Antioxidants: The tropical fruits in this smoothie are a fantastic source of antioxidants, which can reduce oxidative stress and enhance overall health.

Positive Effects on Skin Health: The vitamins and antioxidants in this smoothie can support the maintenance of clear, healthy skin.

Reduces Inflammation: The body's inflammatory reaction may be lessened by the anti-inflammatory properties of several of the components in this smoothie, such as pineapple.

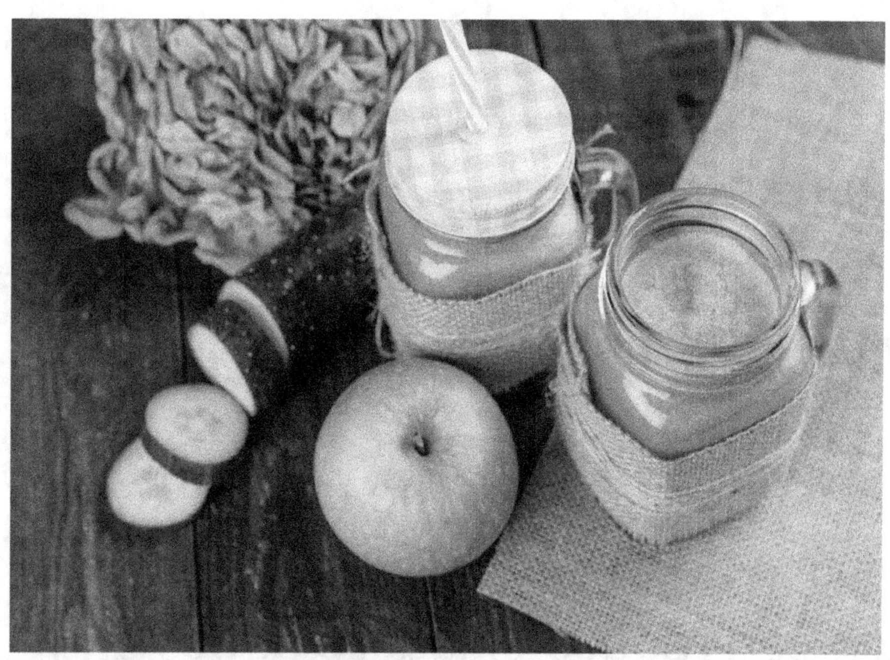

♦ SMOOTHIE WITH GREEN GODDESS

INGREDIENTS:
Water mug.
One scoop of protein powder, optionally vanilla.
A quarter cup fresh baby spinach.
Slicing one celery stalk very thin.
One kiwi, peeled.
One green apple, cored and coarsely sliced.

½ pear, cut into rough pieces after cored.
One small cucumber, sliced and peeled (½).
Roughly cut, peel, and pit a medium avocado.
A dozen or so ice cubes.

INSTRUCTIONS:
Place all the ingredients in a high-speed blender in the specified sequence. Make sure the spinach is totally swamped by the other ingredients to ensure that everything is well blended and there are no big chunks of spinach leaves.

Process until completely smooth, 45–60 seconds at a high speed. Take a sip from a high glass.

NOTES:
When making this green drink for the first time, you may need to taste it and modify as needed. If it's not sweet enough, add a little extra fruit or apple or pineapple juice.

Some smoothies are great to make ahead, but the water content of the cucumber and celery causes this green goddess smoothie to split easily. Drink this immediately while it's still cold for the best mouthfeel.

♦ STRAWBERRY KIWI REFRESHER SMOOTHIE

INGREDIENTS:
Peel and cut into quarters two small, ripe kiwis.
Frozen strawberry chunks, half a cup.
Remove the peel and pith from one clementine or half a medium orange.
Half of a banana, cut and frozen.
Half a cup of your preferred nondairy or skim milk.
Two teaspoons of either regular or quick-cooking rolled oats.
Add a tiny handful of ice to the smoothie if you'd like it thicker and frostier.

Optional: add one to two tsp honey.

INSTRUCTIONS:
Blend together the oats, milk, ice (if using), oranges, strawberries, and kiwis in your blender.

Blend until well combined. Taste and adjust the sweetness with a spoonful or two of honey. Enjoy it now.

Storage Recommendations: Smoothies are best enjoyed immediately upon mixing. Any leftover food should be refrigerated in an airtight jar (the less air, the better) for up to one day. Shake or mix to recombine before serving, and enjoy.

♦ SMOOTHIE WITH MANGO MINT MADNESS

INGREDIENTS.

One cup of mango.

Two green lettuce cups.

Five large mint leaves.

Squeeze half of a lemon.

Half of a lime, juiced.

Just one banana.

A quarter of a cup of unsweetened coconut milk or any other kind of unsweetened milk alternative (almond, cashew, etc.).

INSTRUCTIONS:

1. Place the mint leaves, coconut milk, and lettuce greens in a blender and pulse until smooth.

2. Continue blending in the other ingredients until the mixture reaches the right consistency. Savor the moment.

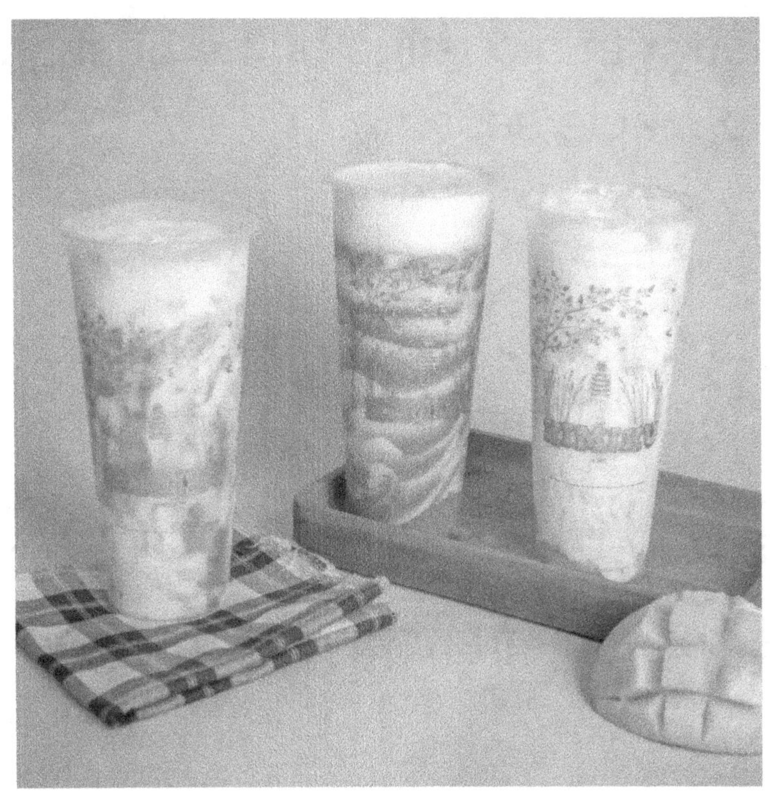

♦ SMOOTHIE WITH CINNAMON APPLE PIE

INGREDIENTS:

One and a half cups of cold paleo cinnamon baked apples.

One cup of plain Greek yogurt, normal or dairy-free.

One third cup of milk, plant-based or not.

Six ice cubes.

One-half tsp of cinnamon.

A sprinkle of sea salt.

Finished with a dusting of the best granola, toasted maple sesame.

INSTRUCTIONS:

In a blender, process all ingredients (excluding granola) until smooth.

Pour into two glasses and sprinkle with the maple sesame granola and spoons!

♦ DELIGHTFUL BLUEBERRY ALMOND SMOOTHIE

INGREDIENTS:

1 cup (my favorite) unsweetened vanilla almond milk.
One peeled banana, either fresh or frozen.
One cup blueberries, either fresh or frozen.
One teaspoon of almond-based butter.
1/3 cup of chia seeds.
A single tablespoon of flaxseed.

INSTRUCTIONS:

Place all the ingredients in a blender and mix until smooth. If you don't use any frozen fruit, you might add a few ice cubes to make it thicker. If your blueberries and banana are frozen, you may need to add a little more almond milk to your blender. Serve immediately.

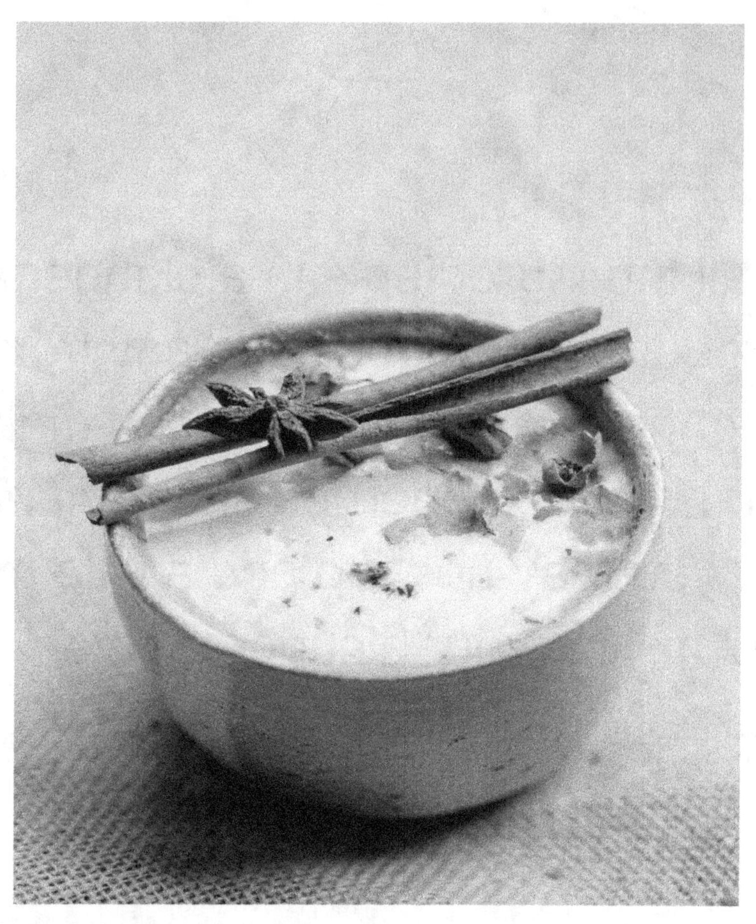

♦ SMOOTHIE WITH VANILLA CHAI SPICE

The ingredient is one scoop of our all-in-one smoothie. Vanilla and Chai.

½ cup vanilla-infused oat milk.

A single cup of ice.

A half-tsp of nutmeg.

A ½ teaspoon of cardamom.

A little salt, please.

A pinch of cinnamon.

Technique of getting ready:
Blend all items together till they are creamy
and smooth.

Transfer to your favorite glass and enjoy!

CHAPTER SEVEN.

Diabetes Friendly Recipes.
(Salad Recipes)

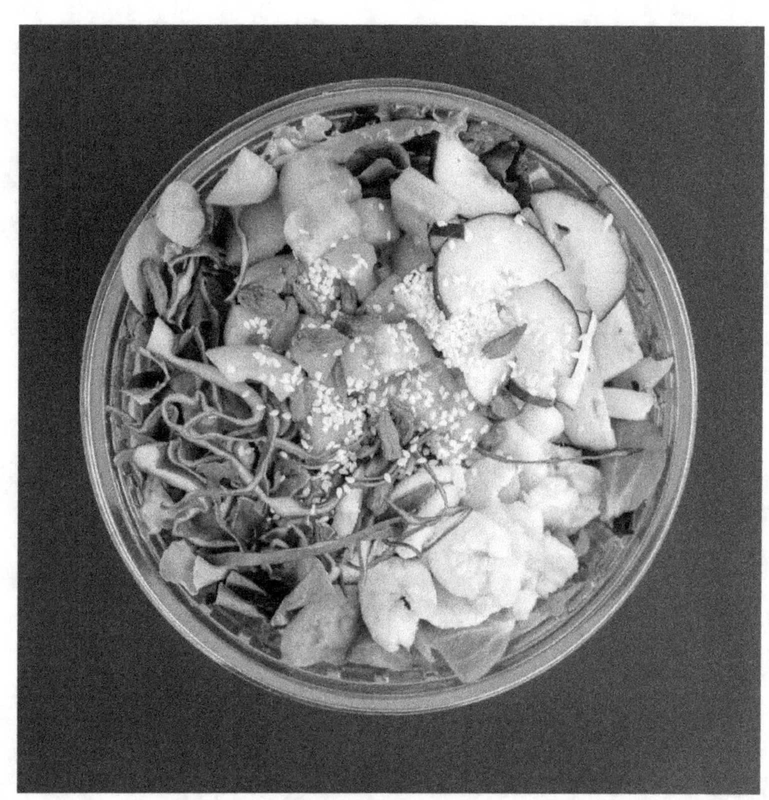

♦ A SALAD WITH ASPARAGUS AND SHRIMP

INGREDIENTS:

One teaspoon of dill seeds.

Olive oil triple-trussed.

Lime juice, two teaspoons.

About 2 tablespoons of finely chopped onion
and One medium shallot.
One teaspoon of mustard dijon.
Sugar, half a teaspoonful.
1/4 teaspoon salt.
One pound of asparagus, trimmed into
2-inch-long pieces and thinly sliced.
One large pound of deveined, skinned shrimp.

INSTRUCTIONS:

In a small pan over medium heat, toast the dill
seeds for one to two minutes, until fragrant.
Remove from the hot pan immediately to avoid
over-toasting.

Using a wire whisk, fully mix the oil, lemon
juice, shallot, mustard, sugar, and salt in a
small bowl. Set aside.

Pour water into a stock pot and heat it until it
boils. When the asparagus is crisp-tender, add
it and boil it for 3 to 4 minutes while stirring.
Using a slotted spoon, swiftly transfer the

asparagus to a dish of cold water to halt the cooking process and allow it to cool. Move to a large bowl and reserve.

Add the shrimp and simmer and refrigerate for a little while longer. Make sure the drain is done correctly. Combine asparagus and shrimp in a big bowl.

Add the shrimp and asparagus to the vinaigrette, being careful to coat well. Serve immediately. Keep chilled and covered until you're ready to serve.

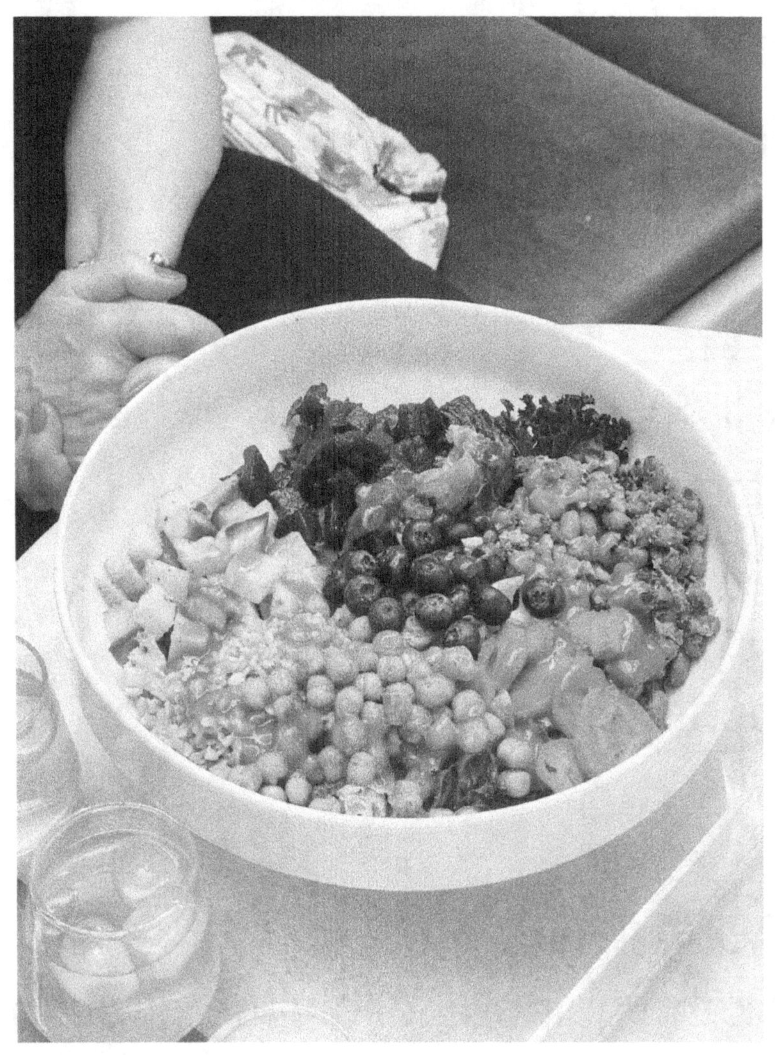

♦ MEDITERRANEAN SALAD WITH QUINOA AND CHICKPEAS

INGREDIENTS:

A cup of uncooked quinoa.

A single can of beans.

A single cup of tomato sauce.

A single cup of cucumbers.

A half-cup carrots.

Just one bell pepper.
Half a red onion.
One bunch of cilantro or parsley.

Dressing:
Olive oil, half a cup.
The juice of one lemon.
Three cloves of garlic.
Salt and pepper.
One-fourth teaspoon dry oregano.

INSTRUCTIONS:
To cook the quinoa, follow the directions on the box. At the end, you should have around two cups of cooked quinoa.

Empty and rinse the chickpeas. Set aside

Chop all the veggies as finely as you can in the interim. Tiny little pieces is the concept here!

In a small bowl, whisk together the oil, lemon juice, minced garlic, salt, pepper, and oregano.

Combine the quinoa, veggies, and chickpeas in a big bowl. Toss to coat with dressing and serve. Potential salad dressing idea: feta cheese

NOTES:

Let the quinoa cool completely first. In heated quinoa, the fresh veggies will wilt. The quinoa may be prepared a day or two ahead of time and kept refrigerated with a lid.

I prefer to make extra dressing to pour over each dish of quinoa while it's still warm, or to drizzle over it.

This salad becomes naturally vegan and dairy-free once the feta is removed. Feel free to add your favorite plant-based feta if you want to enjoy the sour and salty aspects.

◆ TACO SALAD PLANT-BASED

INGREDIENTS:
Olive oil, extra virgin, two tsp.
One large onion, chopped coarsely.
One and a half cups of fresh or frozen corn kernels (see Tip).
Four large tomatoes.
Steamed one and a half cups long-grain brown rice (see tip).
One fifteen-ounce can of rinsed pinto or black kidney beans.
A single teaspoon of chili powder.
One-half teaspoon dried oregano, divided.
Half a teaspoon of salt.
1/4 cup of finely chopped fresh cilantro.
A third cup of salsa is ready.
Two cups of finely chopped iceberg or romaine lettuce.
Shredded pepper Jack cheese (one cup).
Two and a half cups of tortilla chips, broken up fine.

Lime slices as a finishing touch.

INSTRUCTIONS:
Add oil to a large nonstick pan and set it over medium heat. Add the onion and corn and cook, stirring, until the onion begins to brown, about 5 minutes. Dice a tomato finely. Add the rice, beans, 1/4 tsp salt, 1 tsp oregano, and chili powder, and toss to coat. Cook, stirring frequently, until the tomato is cooked through, about 5 minutes. Let it cool down a bit.

Roughly chop the final three tomatoes. Combine the salsa, cilantro, and the last 1/2 teaspoon of oregano in a medium-sized bowl.

In a big bowl, mix together the lettuce, bean mixture, 2/3 cup of cheese, and half of the fresh salsa. Arrange lime wedges and any remaining fresh salsa on the table; sprinkle the remaining cheese and tortilla chips on top.

Plan ahead and prepare as directed in Step 1, cover, and refrigerate for up to 3 days. Just reheat until ready to serve.

To extract the corn from the cob, hold the corn ear by its stem end and use a sharp knife to chop off the kernels.

Bring one cup of water and half a cup of long-grain brown rice to a boil in a small pot. Lower the heat to low, cover, and cook the rice for approximately 40 minutes, or until it is tender and the water has been absorbed. Once the heat is off, cover and let sit for 10 minutes. Produces half a cup.

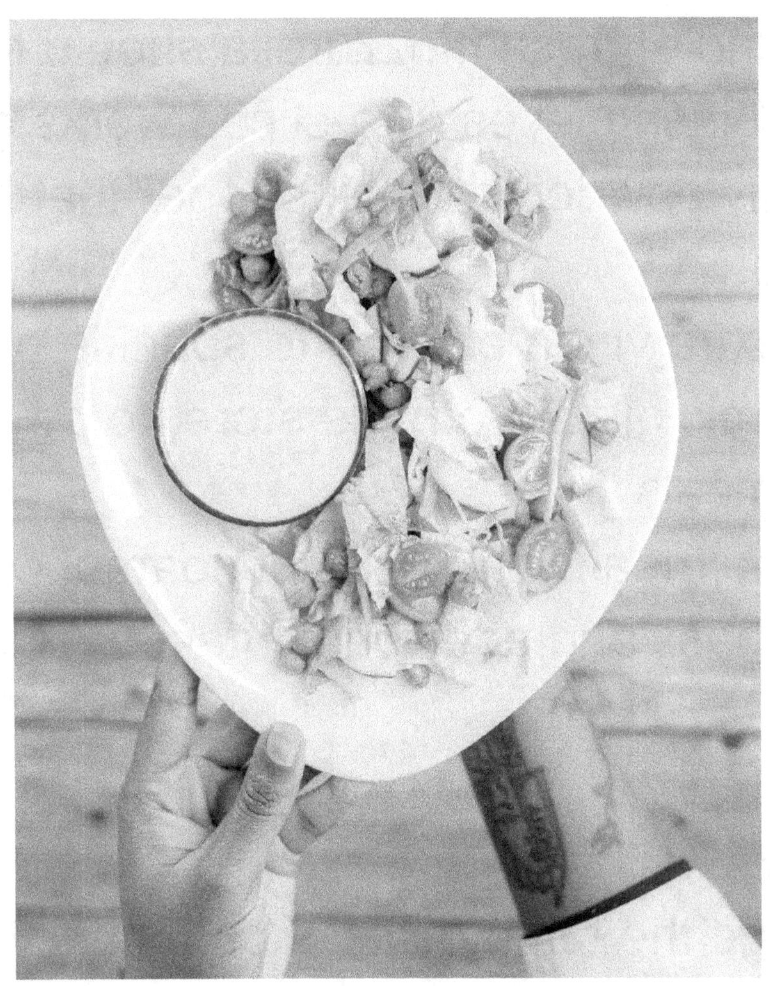

♦ A SALAD DRESSED WITH BALSAMIC GLAZE

INGREDIENTS:

Three heirloom or vine-ripened tomatoes, cut into ¼-inch slices.
Half a teaspoon of sweetener.
Cut the ½ teaspoon of salt in half.

A pound of fresh mozzarella should be sliced into ¼-inch pieces (pre-sliced works good too).

Freshly powdered black pepper that has been tasted.

Use extra virgin olive oil to sprinkle over food.

Balsamic glaze from the store, to be drizzled over meals.

Top the meal with ¼ cup of coarsely chopped fresh basil and additional intact basil sprigs.

INSTRUCTIONS:

Arrange the tomato slices on a cutting surface. In order to dissolve the sugar, add a tsp of salt and sugar and let it sit for a few minutes.

Arrange the mozzarella and tomato slices one after the other on a platter. Use the remaining ¼ teaspoon of salt and freshly ground black pepper to season evenly. Drizzle a tablespoon of olive oil and the same amount of balsamic glaze on top (you can just eyeball it). Among them, distribute the finely chopped basil.

Garnish the meal with fresh basil leaves, if desired.

♦ A SALAD WITH SPINACH AND STRAWBERRIES

INGREDIENTS:
Olive oil, extra virgin, two tsp.
A tablespoon of white balsamic vinegar should be taken.
Add coarse salt and freshly ground pepper.
Four cups of softly packed baby spinach.
Six ounces (1 ½ cups) of hulled strawberries, thinly sliced.
1/4 cup of roasted almonds, chopped coarsely (1 ½ ounces).
A tablespoon of sesame seeds, toasted.
Two ounces of feta in crumbles.

In a large basin, whisk together the vinegar and oil. For seasoning, add salt and pepper. Incorporate the feta, spinach, sesame seeds, strawberries, and almonds. Gently toss the spinach until the dressing is evenly incorporated. Serve immediately.

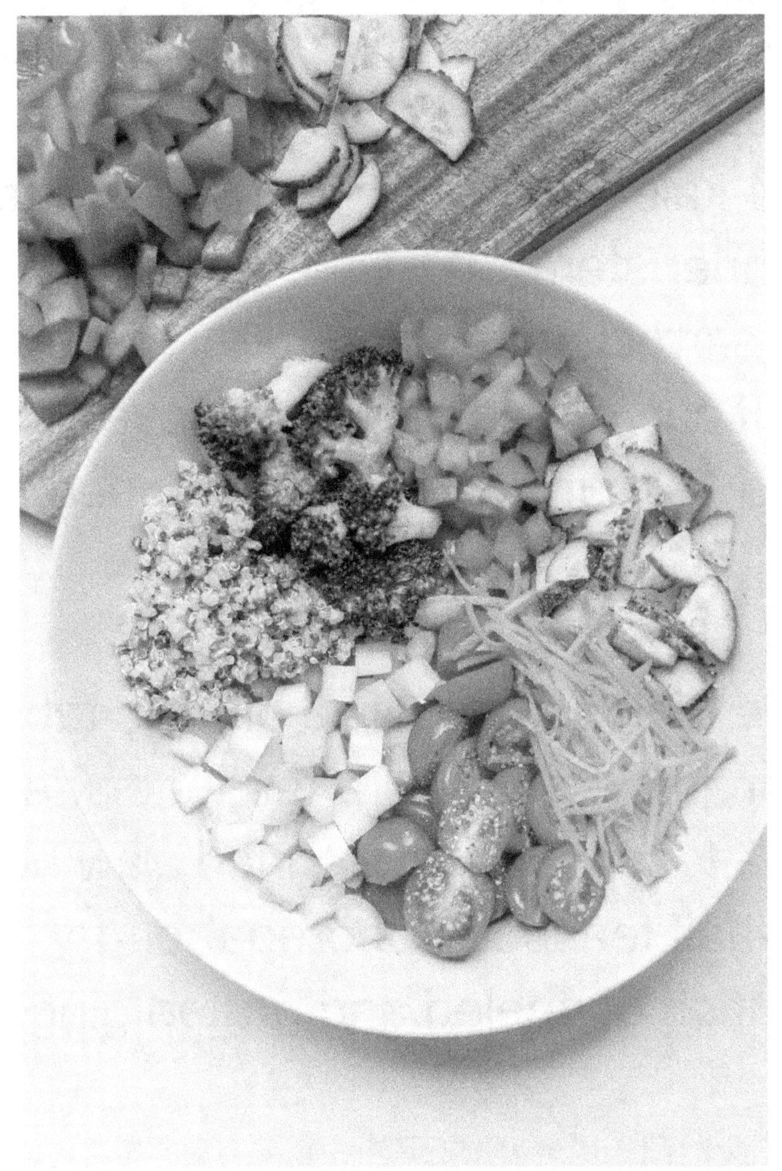

♦ DETOX SALAD WITH CAULIFLOWER AND BROCCOLI.

FOR THE SALAD:

One head of broccoli yields around 2 1/2 cups of finely chopped broccoli.

Cut up half a head (two cups) of cauliflower into small pieces.
Cut 4 kale leaves into thin slices after removing the inner stem.
Two carrots, shreds.
A half cup of fresh parsley leaves, cut just now.
1/4 to 1/2 cup of walnuts, chopped finely.

FOR THE DRESSING:

Three tablespoons olive oil, two tablespoons lemon juice, and half a teaspoon zest.
Half a teaspoon of unrefined, raw honey.
One-half teaspoon of oregano, dry.
One inch of peeled and grated ginger.

INSTRUCTIONS:

Combine all the dressing ingredients in a small bowl and keep it ready.
In a large bowl, add all salad ingredients and whisk to mix.
Pour dressing over all of the ingredients and stir until well combined and lightly covered.

Store in the fridge in an airtight container for up to 3 days.

♦ GREEK COUSCOUS SALAD.

INGREDIENTS:
For the salad, use one fifteen-ounce can of rinsed and drained chickpeas.
Dice one bell pepper, red.
Chop one bell pepper, yellow.
Dice one bell pepper, green.
1/4 cup finely sliced red onion.
About one cup of halved grape tomatoes, or fifteen half-grape tomatoes.
If desired, add one-third cup chopped, pitted Kalamata olives.
Halve a medium cucumber lengthwise.
Four ounces of feta cheese, crumbled or cut into half-inch pieces.
Putting on clothes.
A couple of tsp olive oil.

Two tablespoons of recently squeezed lemon juice.
One clove of minced garlic.
One teaspoon of dried oregano.
Season to taste with freshly ground pepper and salt.

INSTRUCTIONS:
Combine all salad ingredients in a large bowl and toss to combine.

Garlic, oregano, lemon juice, and olive oil should all be combined in a small bowl. Pour over the salad and give it another good stir. Taste and adjust with extra salt and pepper as needed.

You may marinate it in the refrigerator for an hour or serve it immediately. Salad should be consumed two to three days after cooking.

Remarks Regarding the Recipe:

I recommend double the ingredients for this salad if you're serving a large crowd! You can even prepare the salad 1-2 days ahead of time because the veggies will marinate deliciously in the dressing.

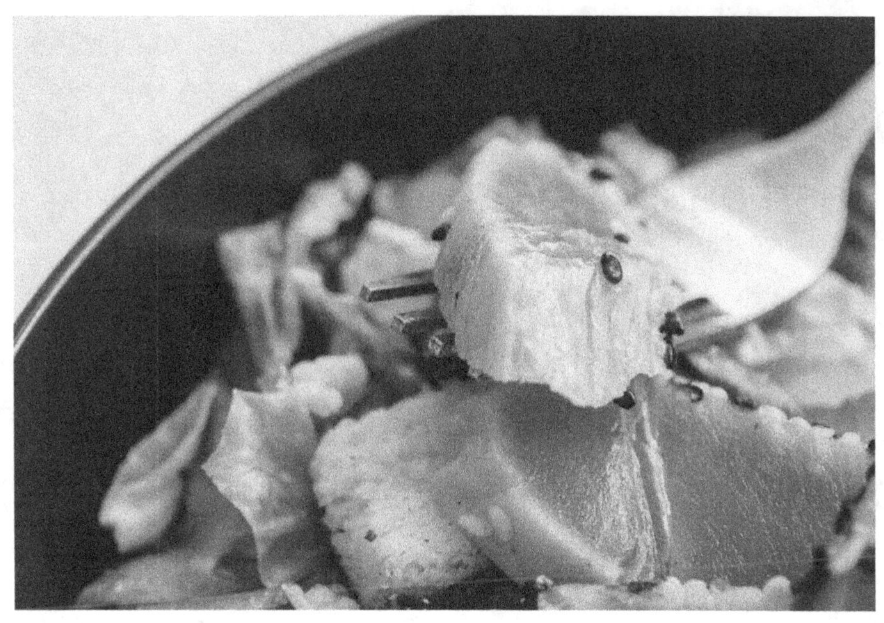

♦ WHITE BEAN SALAD WITH TUNA.

INGREDIENTS:

Two 6-oz cans of tuna with dark meat and plenty of olive oil.

Cannellini white beans, drained and cleaned, in two 15-ounce cans.

One-third cup small capers, rinsed and drained, not brined pareil.

A half-cup vinegar made from red wine.

Black pepper that has just been ground and sea salt.

Thinly slice one medium red onion.

1 1/2 cups cherry tomatoes.

Two cups of uncooked arugula.

Six fresh basil leaves.

INSTRUCTIONS:

Empty the olive oil into a smaller bowl and place the tuna in the larger one. Cut the tuna into bite-sized pieces using a large fork. Add the beans and capers. Transfer the red wine vinegar to the olive oil basin. The suggested ratio is one part vinegar to two parts oil; add extra virgin olive oil as needed. For seasoning, add salt and pepper. Drizzle the dressing over the tuna, bean, and caper mixture and allow the flavors to permeate while you cut the

vegetables. With caution, toss in the tomatoes
and onion with the tuna mixture.
Spoon the tuna mixture over the arugula in a
big decorative plate. Tear fresh basil leaves,
then serve immediately.

CHAPTER EIGHT.

Diabetes Friendly Recipes.
(Bonus Recipes)
A. APPETIZER RECIPES.

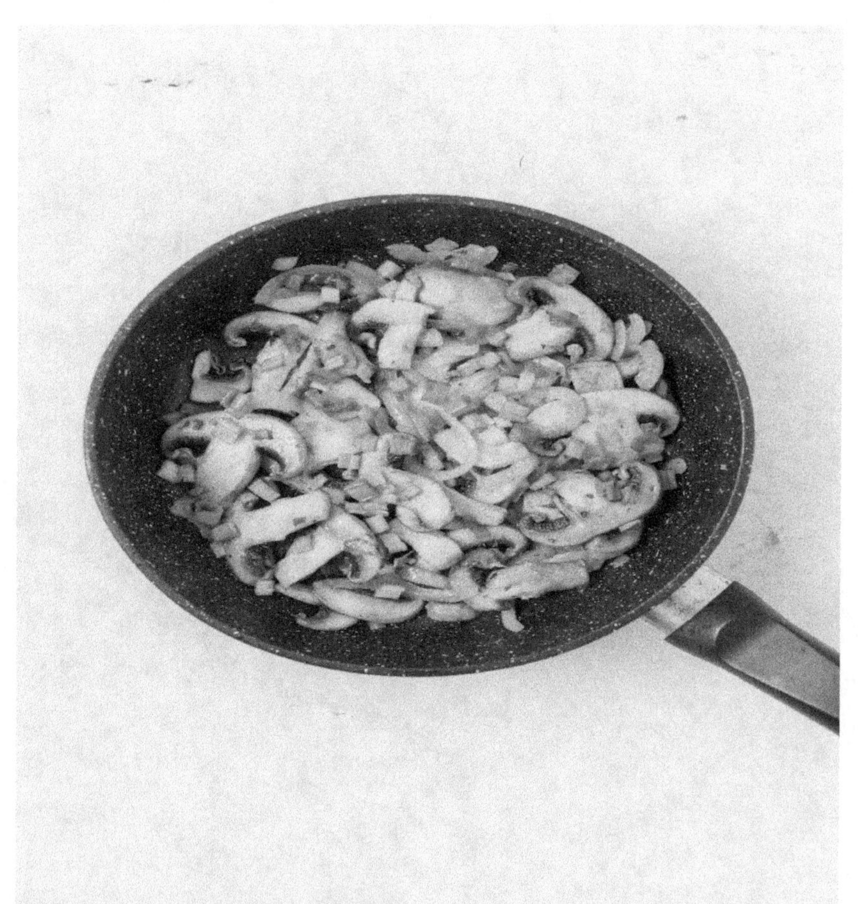

♦ STUFFED SPINACH FETA MUSHROOMS

INGREDIENTS:

One tablespoon of extra virgin olive oil.
Two cups (sixty grams) of fresh spinach,
packed.
100 grams, or 3.5 ounces, of feta cheese.
one clove of garlic.
Twelve button mushrooms.

INSTRUCTIONS:

Set the oven's temperature to 400°F (200°C).

The oil should be heated in a skillet or frying
pan. Pressed garlic is added after a minute or
so of sautéing the spinach. For one another
minute or until the spinach has totally wilted,
stir regularly. Take off the heat source.

Use a moist towel to wipe the mushrooms
clean, or remove their skin.

Using a fork, mix the crumbled feta and
sautéed spinach in a small bowl.

Place approximately one spoonful of the filling inside each mushroom. Transfer them to a baking pan and bake for 20 minutes, or until done, at 400°F/200°C.

Serve either cold or warm.

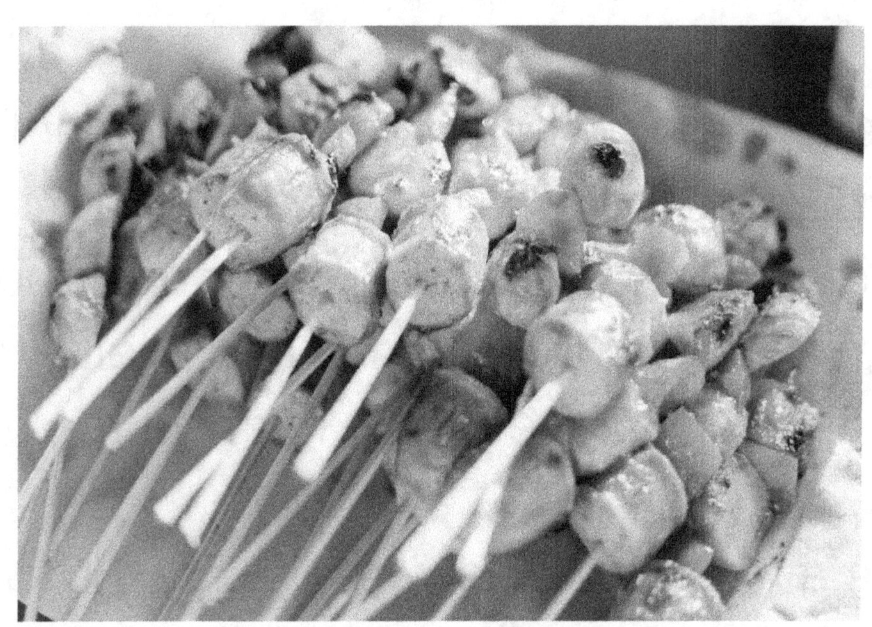

♦ SKEWERS OF GRILLED SHRIMP

INGREDIENTS:
A one pound of large, deveined, peeled shrimp

Two tablespoons lemon juice and three
tablespoons olive oil
A half-tsp each of black pepper and salt
One teaspoon of oregano
one-half teaspoon paprika
One-half teaspoon of powdered garlic
chopped parsley for the dish
Slices of lemon for serving

INSTRUCTIONS:
In a large bowl, add the olive oil, lemon juice,
garlic powder, oregano, paprika, salt, and
pepper. Whisk to mix.

Toss the shrimp lightly in the dish to ensure
that they are equally coated with marinade.
Marinate for a minimum of 15 minutes and a
maximum of 2 hours.

While skewering the remaining shrimp, skewer
four to six of them at a time and set them aside
on a plate.

When the grill or grill pan is hot, add the shrimp and cook them for two to three minutes on each side, or until they are opaque and pink in color.

If preferred, garnish warm servings with lemon slices and fresh parsley.

♦ BAKED ZUCCHINI CHIPS

INGREDIENTS:
Spray with olive oil.
Two medium zucchini, weighing a combined one pound.
1 ¼ teaspoon salt ½ teaspoon garlic powder.
A tsp of black pepper.
¼ cup grated (not shredded) parmesan cheese.

GUIDELINES:

Set oven temperature to 425°F. Grease a rimmed baking sheet with olive oil spray and line it with high-heat-resistant parchment paper.

Cut the zucchini into rounds that are ⅛ inch thick. Apply a single teaspoon of kosher salt to each slice. After putting the salted zucchini in a sink colander, let it rest at room temperature for half an hour. This ought to extract some of the water. Slices of zucchini should be rinsed and blotted dry with paper towels after 30 minutes.

On the baking sheet that has been prepared, arrange the zucchini slices in a single layer. Apply a little layer of olive oil on them. For fifteen minutes, bake them.

Take out of the oven the baking sheet. Add the remaining ¼ teaspoon of kosher salt, black pepper, garlic powder, and grated Parmesan cheese to the zucchini pieces. The zucchini don't need to be flipped.

Put the pan back in the oven and bake for a further 15 to 20 minutes, or until the zucchini slices are crisp and golden.

♦ CAULIFLOWER HUMMUS

INGREDIENTS:

5 cups (14–15 ounces) of cauliflower florets.
1 huge clove minced garlic.
1 3/4 tsp finely ground kosher salt, split.
Half a cup of sesame tahini.
Add extra virgin olive oil (about 1/3 cup) for serving.
three teaspoons of lemon juice.
Finely chopped sumac and parsley to serve.

INSTRUCTIONS:

1. In a pot with a steamer attachment, bring an inch of water to a boil. When the cauliflower is

extremely soft when probed with a fork, add it and simmer it covered for about 6 minutes.

2. In the meantime, add one teaspoon of salt to the garlic and crush it with the side of the knife until a paste forms.

3. Attach the steel blade to the food processor. To chop up the cauliflower, add the cauliflower and garlic salt, then pulse a few times.

4. Crack open the cover and add the lemon, tahini, olive oil, and the remaining ¾ teaspoon of salt. Cover and carry out. Process the cauliflower, scraping down the sides, until it's extremely smooth and has the consistency of soft hummus.

5. Spoon onto a platter for serving. For about two hours, or until cool and hard, cover and refrigerate. Pour in a little more olive oil. Before serving, top with sumac and parsley.

◆ VEGGIE PLATTER ON THE GRILL WITH YOGURT-MINT SAUCE

INGREDIENTS:

One cup of Greek yogurt (0%).

Partition 1/4 cup of newly chopped mint.

Two garlic cloves, chopped and split.

One teaspoon each of salt, black pepper, and extra virgin olive oil.

VEGETABLES:

2 big bell peppers, red and orange in hue, seeded and chopped into 1-inch pieces.

One red onion, cut into rounds about 1/4 inch thick.

One pound of cleaned asparagus.

One yellow squash, cut into 1/4-inch-thick diagonal slices.

One big zucchini, cut into 1/4-inch-thick diagonal slices.

Two tablespoons of premium virgin olive oil.

two tsp lemon juice.

One teaspoon of Zataar seasoning, dry.

One-half tsp salt.

One-fourth teaspoon of pepper.

INSTRUCTIONS:

Mix yogurt with 1/4 teaspoon salt, black pepper, half of the mint, and half of the garlic. Move to a little serving dish. Drizzle with a teaspoon of olive oil and add more mint as a garnish.

Turn the heat up to medium-high on the grill or grill pan. Once prepared, oil the grilles.

In a bowl, combine the veggies, zaatar, lemon juice, olive oil, 1/2 teaspoon salt, and black pepper, according to taste. The veggies should be mildly browned after 6 to 10 minutes of grilling, with periodic flipping. Place with the mint yogurt sauce on a plate. Add the remaining mint on top.

B. PORK RECIPES.

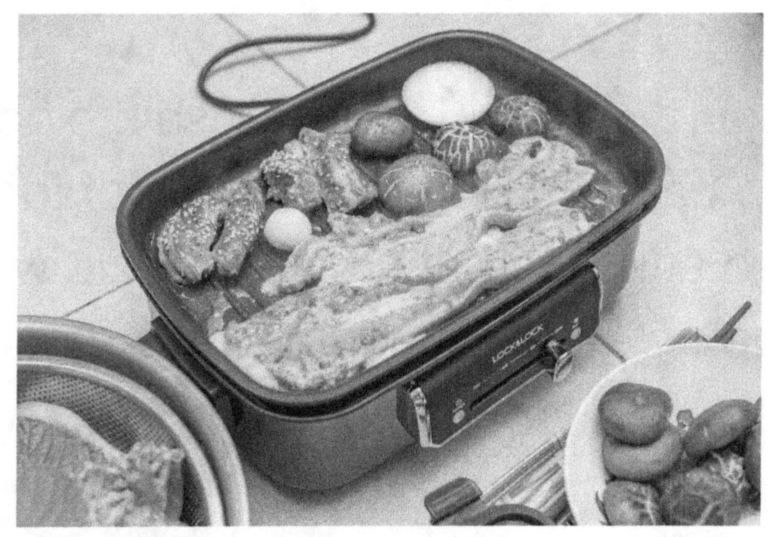

♦ MUSHROOM AND SPINACH STUFFED PORK LOIN

INGREDIENTS:

Split two teaspoons of olive oil.
1/4 pound of coarsely chopped mushrooms.

six to eight cups of finely chopped, raw spinach
One little bag.
three garlic cloves.
one-half teaspoon of thyme.
Half a spoonful of soy sauce.
One-third cup cream cheese.
One-half cup Panko bread crumbs.
One 1.5-pound pork tenderloin.
One spoonful of mustard dijon.
Add the salt and pepper.

INSTRUCTIONS:

Turn the oven on to 450°F.

In a pan, heat up one tablespoon of olive oil.
Add the mushrooms, soy sauce, and garlic,
and simmer for approximately 5 minutes, or
until the mushrooms are softened. The liquid
from the mushrooms helps keep the lean pork
moist.

Cook the chopped spinach until it wilts. Take off the heat and whisk in the panko crumbs, cream cheese, and thyme.

Refrigerate the filling until it cools completely.

PORK TENDERLOIN:
Slice the pork tenderloin in half lengthwise, but do not cut it open; this will make the meat butterfly-shaped.

Once the pork is uniformly thick, approximately ½ inch, pound it.

Cover the pork with the cooled filling, roll it like a jelly roll, and fasten it with toothpicks.

Brush tenderloin with a mixture of dijon and one tablespoon olive oil. Add pepper and salt for seasoning.

Bake until the temperature hits 135°F, about 25 to 30 minutes.

Once browned and the internal temperature reaches 145°F, broil for an additional five minutes.

Give it a five-minute rest before cutting.

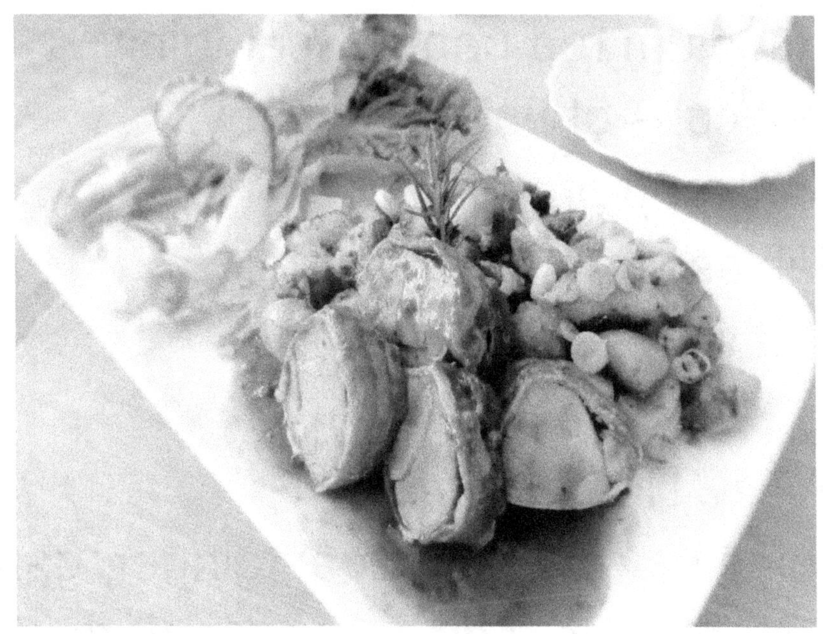

♦ VEGETABLE STIR-FRY WITH PORK AND VEGGIES

One pound of boneless pork tenderloin that has been thinly sliced and fattened.
1/4 cup of soy sauce.

Two tablespoons of brown sugar.
two minced garlic cloves.
Two teaspoons of freshly peeled and coarsely
sliced ginger.
1/4 teaspoon crushed red pepper.
One tablespoon of canola oil.
3 julienne medium carrots.
1 and a half cups broccoli stems.
One medium red pepper, cut thinly.
Chop 2 cups of baby bok choy.
One-half cup orange juice.
two tablespoons cornstarch.
garnish with sesame seeds.

INSTRUCTIONS:
Combine soy sauce, sugar, ginger, garlic, and
pepper flakes in a dish. Toss in pork strips;
cover and marinate for half an hour.

In a nonstick skillet, heat the oil over high heat.
Save the marinade after removing the pork
pieces from it. After cooking the pork strips for
three to four minutes, remove and set aside.

Stir in the broccoli and carrots and simmer for 2 minutes, or until the vegetables are starting to soften. If the pan seems dry, add 2 Tbsp/30 mL of orange juice. Stir-fry the red pepper and bok choy for two minutes, or until they are crisp-tender.

Mix cornstarch and orange juice in a small dish.

After marinating, return the pork strips to the skillet along with the orange juice. Stir-fry until sauce thickens, approximately 1 minute. Accompany with noodles or rice.

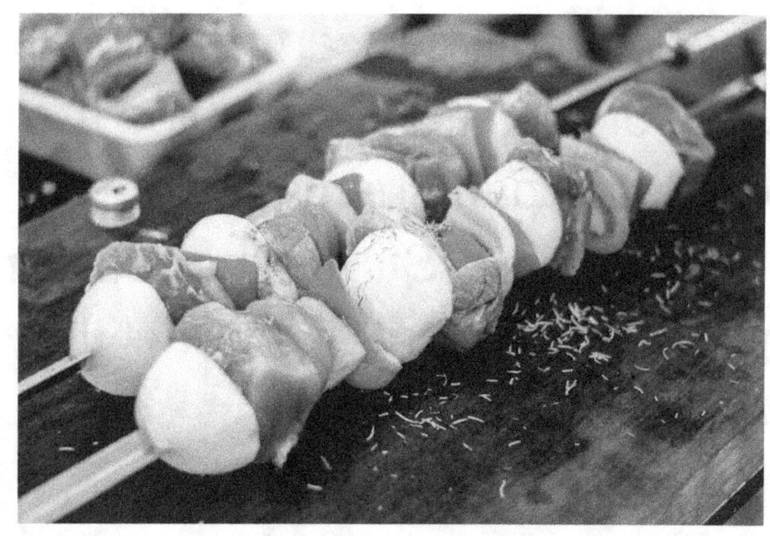

♦ PORK CHOPS GLAZED WITH APPLE CIDER

FOR THE PORK CHOPS:

Pork loin chops, boneless, weighing 1 1/2 pounds.

pepper and salt.

1/2 teaspoon powdered garlic.

Half a teaspoon of chili powder.

two tablespoons all-purpose flour.

Two tablespoons of oil.

FOR THE GLAZE:

One cup of cider apple.

Apple cider vinegar, one tablespoon.

Two tablespoons of honey.
One teaspoon Dijon mustard.
Add pepper and salt to taste.

INSTRUCTIONS:

After using a paper towel to pat the pork chops dry, season them with salt and pepper on both sides. Garlic powder, chili powder, and flour should all be thoroughly mixed in a small basin.

After dusting each pork chop with seasoned flour, pat it to ensure uniform coating. Put the pork chops aside so that the flour can absorb the liquid they emit.

Heat a sizable skillet over medium-high heat and let it cook through evenly. After adding the oil, carefully fit as many pork chops onto the skillet as possible without packing it too full.

Cook until the first side is a deep golden brown, about 2-3 minutes. Then, turn it over and continue cooking for another 1-2 minutes, depending on thickness, or until the second side is cooked through but still somewhat raw. Place the pork chops on a platter, gently tent with aluminum foil, and keep it covered.

Put the skillet back on the burner and whisk together the apple cider, vinegar, honey, and Dijon. As you raise the liquid to a boil, make sure all of the brown particles are dissolved into the cider by scraping down the pan's bottom.

Boil the liquid quickly for 7-8 minutes, or until it thickens and reduces by a little more than half. After removing from the fire, add salt and pepper to taste in the glaze. Serve the pork chops right away by covering them with glaze or by returning them to the skillet and rotating them to coat them.

◆ PULL PORK LETTUCE WRAPS WITH LOW-CARB AND SLOW COOKER RECIPES

INGREDIENTS:

Pork shoulder, 2 pounds.

Two teaspoons of onion powder.

1 teaspoon powdered garlic.

Two teaspoons of dried rosemary.

Two tsp. of paprika smoked.

One-half teaspoon cayenne powder.

One teaspoon of powdered fennel seeds.

Two teaspoons of cocoa powder.

To taste, add salt and black pepper.

Half a cup chicken stock.

Eight leaves of butter lettuce or iceberg.

INSTRUCTIONS:

In a small dish, mix together all the spices and cocoa; add salt and black pepper to taste. After giving the pork shoulder a thorough coat of spice, place it in a 5- or 6-quart slow cooker pot. Put the chicken broth in the crock pot and simmer for four hours on high or six hours on low heat.

When the cooking time is up, take the pork out of the slow cooker crock and shred it with two forks. To enhance the taste, let the pulled pork sit in the juices for 20 to 30 minutes while keeping the slow cooker on "warm."

When ready to serve, place some crisp broccoli slaw inside each lettuce leaf and top with pulled pork. Have fun!

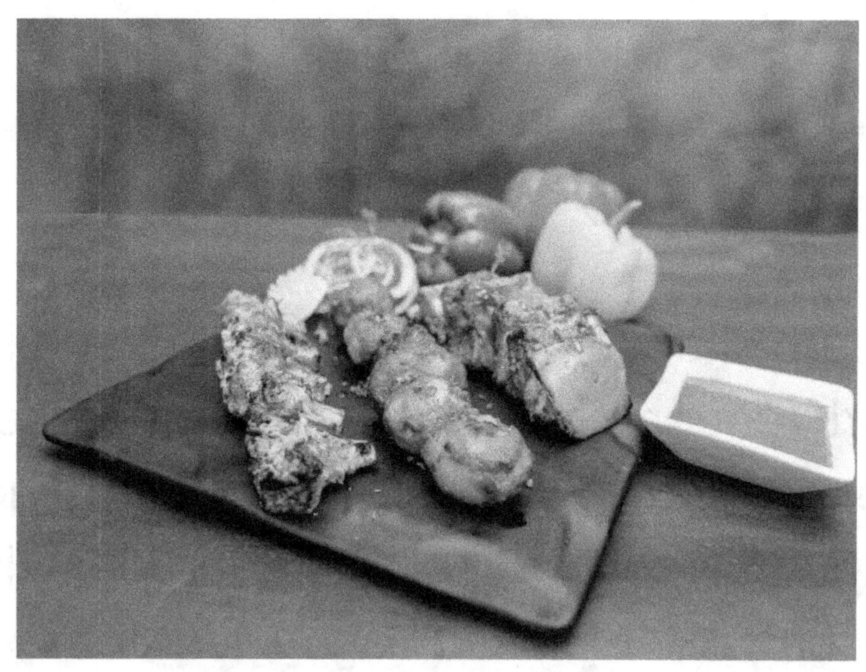

◆ GRILLED PORK TENDERLOIN WITH LEMON AND GARLIC AND CHARRED GREEN BEANS

INGREDIENTS:

Two whole, nearly two-pound pork tenderloins, with the silver skin removed and trimmed.

Zest and juice two huge, juicy lemons.

Eight garlic cloves, minced or grated coarsely.

1/4 cup finely chopped fresh, hardy herbs, such thyme, sage, rosemary, or oregano.

Three tablespoons of extra virgin olive oil.

Two teaspoons of mustard dijon.

One spoonful of honey.

To season, add kosher salt, ground black pepper, or crushed red chili flakes.

INSTRUCTIONS:

Ready the lemon-herb marinade and let the pork tenderloin sit in it: Transfer the garlic, fresh herbs, olive oil, Dijon mustard, honey, lemon zest and juice, and a large baking dish or resealable plastic bag. Add 2 teaspoons of kosher salt, ground black pepper, and crushed red chili flakes for seasoning, if preferred. Mix by whisking.

Toss the pork tenderloin in the baking dish to ensure that the marinade of lemon and herbs is all over it. Put the lid on and let it marinate for six to twelve hours.

Warm up the grill. Take the pork tenderloin out of the refrigerator 30 minutes before you want to start grilling so it can come to room temperature while the grill heats up. Get the grill ready for direct heat cooking at 500–550 degrees Fahrenheit.

Shake off any extra marinade into the baking dish before placing the marinated pork tenderloin on the grill so that it is perpendicular to the grill grates. Throw away extra marinade. Once an instant-read thermometer placed in the center of the pork tenderloin registers an internal temperature of 145 degrees F, close the cover and grill the pork tenderloin for 10 to 12 minutes, flipping it every 3 to 4 minutes to achieve uniform cooking. Move the tenderloin of pork to a large dish or serving tray. Before serving, tent with foil and let it a three-minute rest.

After the pork tenderloin has rested, serve it. Cut into 1/2-inch-thick medallions and serve with your preferred summertime sides (the charred green beans in the recipe are shown). Have fun!

CONCLUSIONS.

As we wrap up the culinary exploration within "Diabetes Balanced Diets," let the essence linger—a lively symphony of flavors that rethink diabetes management. This book isn't just about recipes; it's a guide leading towards a life where every meal is a celebration of health and joy. To all the readers and people handling diabetes, remember that each mindful choice is a step towards informed well-being. Embrace the richness of balanced living, revel in the delicious possibilities, and let every bite be a statement that managing diabetes can be both tasty and satisfying. This journey doesn't end with the last page—it continues with each healthy meal. Cheers to a life where wellness is a delightful, ongoing adventure, and to the triumphs of accepting a balanced and delicious way forward.

REVIEWS.

Dear Valued Readers,

I trust this message finds you well. We sincerely appreciate your support in choosing "Diabetes Balanced Diets." Your commitment to a healthier lifestyle is truly commendable.

As we strive to enhance our future publications, we kindly request a few moments of your time to share your valuable feedback. Your insights and opinions on the book would be immensely beneficial in shaping our future endeavors and ensuring we continue to meet your expectations.

If you could spare a moment to leave a review on the platform where you purchased the book, we would be truly grateful. Your honest thoughts on the content, presentation, and any suggestions for improvement will contribute significantly to our ongoing commitment to providing high-quality resources for those managing diabetes.

We deeply appreciate your time and thoughtful consideration. Thank you for being a part of our journey towards better health and well-being.

Warm regards,
Dr. Neal Allan.